Bud Werner Memorial Library
1289 Lincoln Ave.
Steamboat Springs, CO 80487
970.879.0240
Renew: www.steamboatlibrary.org

0817

D1016955

More Advance Praise for *Open Heart*

"Westaby is everything you would hope from a maverick surgical genius: authoritative, engaged, passionate and opinionated. His book, annoyingly well written for someone who has penned only medical papers and handbooks, reads like a thriller, except with rather more corpses. You race to each chapter's end to see if his certain-to-die patient survives."
—*The Times*

"In his powerful book, Westaby tells how the 'back-street boy' from a Scunthorpe housing estate decided to become a heart surgeon."
—*The Observer*

"A full-frontal and thrilling portrayal. Each story in this fascinating book brings a new nail-biting surgical adventure . . . A gifted surgeon, Westaby is also a natural writer . . . [*Open Heart*] succeeds on many levels: political battle cry, chronicle of bloody feats, history of modern cardiology, tribute to patients and paean to surgery."
—*The Daily Telegraph*

"Profoundly powerful . . . Writing with a brisk, brash style, Westaby details the lives of his patients and their operations with precision, gusto, and humour."
—*The Literary Review*

"At the cutting-edge of scalpel-lit . . . I love getting a window into this world . . . I enjoyed so much in this book—the anatomy lesson, the vivid descriptions, the fervour Westaby feels for his work."
—*The Evening Standard*

"Remarkable."
—*The Daily Mirror*

OPEN
HEART

OPEN
HEART

A Cardiac Surgeon's Stories *of*
Life *and* Death *on the* Operating Table

Stephen Westaby

BASIC BOOKS
NEW YORK

Copyright © 2017 by Stephen Westaby
Published by Basic Books, an imprint of Perseus Books, LLC, a subsidiary of
Hachette Book Group, Inc.

All rights reserved. Printed in the United States of America. No part of this book
may be reproduced in any manner whatsoever without written permission except in
the case of brief quotations embodied in critical articles and reviews. For information, address Basic Books, 1290 Avenue of the Americas, New York, NY 10104.

Books published by Basic Books are available at special discounts for bulk purchases
in the United States by corporations, institutions, and other organizations. For more
information, please contact the Special Markets Department at Perseus Books, 2300
Chestnut Street, Suite 200, Philadelphia, PA 19103, or call (800) 810-4145, ext. 5000,
or e-mail special.markets@perseusbooks.com.

DESIGNED BY LINDA MARK

Library of Congress Cataloging-in-Publication Data
Names: Westaby, Stephen, author.
Title: Open heart : a cardiac surgeon's stories of life and death on the
    operating table / Stephen Westaby.
Description: New York : Basic Books, [2017] | Includes index.
Identifiers: LCCN 2016058151 (print) | LCCN 2016059363 (ebook) |
    ISBN 9780465094837 (hardcover) | ISBN 9780465094844 (ebook)
Subjects: | MESH: Cardiac Surgical Procedures | Cardiologists | Personal Narratives
Classification: LCC RD598 (print) | LCC RD598 (ebook) | NLM WG 168 | DDC
    617.4/12—dc23
LC record available at https://lccn.loc.gov/2016058151

LSC-C

10 9 8 7 6 5 4 3 2 1

To my wonderful children, Gemma and Mark,
and granddaughters, Alice and Chloe

Contents

Prologue

WOODY ALLEN FAMOUSLY SAID, "MY BRAIN: IT'S MY second-favorite organ." I had the same affinity with the heart. Well, other people's hearts. I liked to watch them. Stop them. Repair them and start them up again. Like a mechanic tinkering beneath the hood of a car. When I finally understood how the heart worked, the rest just followed. After all, in my younger days, I had been an artist. Both painting and heart surgery required precision and fine motor skills. I simply shifted from brush on canvas to scalpel on human flesh. More hobby than job. More pleasure than chore. It was something I was good at.

The heart had a pleasing symmetry to it, or at least I thought it did, initially. My school biology classes described it as an organ of four parts. Two collecting chambers, the left and right atrium, and two pumping chambers, the left and right ventricle. Textbook diagrams show the atria and ventricles side by side. Like a house with two compact bedrooms, situated above a spacious sitting room and

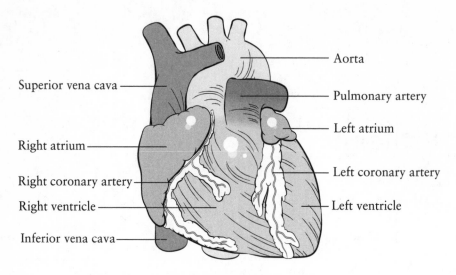

Superior vena cava

Right atrium

Right coronary artery

Right ventricle

Inferior vena cava

Aorta

Pulmonary artery

Left atrium

Left coronary artery

Left ventricle

Heart Anterior

kitchen. The spongy, expansible lungs surround the heart, resembling the steeply pitched roof of an A-frame. The lungs continuously replenish blood oxygen levels and expel carbon dioxide and other chemicals into the atmosphere.

But is it all really that simple? My mother used to buy sheep hearts from the butcher. Inexpensive and tasty enough. Great for dissecting. It was then that I discovered that real hearts are more complex and idiosyncratic than the diagrams showed. Fundamentally, the shape and muscular architecture of the two ventricles are very different. Nor are they left and right. More front and back. The thicker left ventricle is conical in shape. It has circular muscle bands that constrict and rotate the chamber. Now we can visualize how the left ventricle really works. As the powerful muscle contracts and thickens (the systolic phase), its cavity narrows and shortens to expel blood through the aortic valve. Then during the heart's filling phase, or diastole, the left ventricle recoils and the aortic valve closes. The recoiling cavity widens and lengthens, sucking blood from the atrium

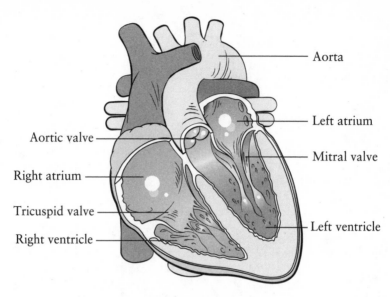

Aorta

Left atrium

Aortic valve

Mitral valve

Right atrium

Tricuspid valve

Left ventricle

Right ventricle

Heart Mitral Valve

into the ventricle through the mitral valve (so named for its likeness to the bishop's miter). During systole, the mitral valve closes again and the contents of the left ventricle are pushed onward around the aorta and the arteries of the body. Thus every coordinated cycle of contraction and relaxation involves narrowing, twisting, and short-ening, followed by widening, uncoiling, and lengthening. A veritable Argentine tango, but with one difference. The whole process takes less than one second and the dance goes on for our entire lives.

Intriguingly, the right ventricle works in an entirely differ-ent way. Situated at the front of the heart between tricuspid and pulmonary valves, it is crescentic in shape and applied to the side of the left ventricle known as the interventricular septum. With this "new moon" shape, the right ventricle pumps like a bellows. The transverse free-wall fibers work against the powerful oblique muscle bonds of the septum—like lovers twisting and coiling their bodies.

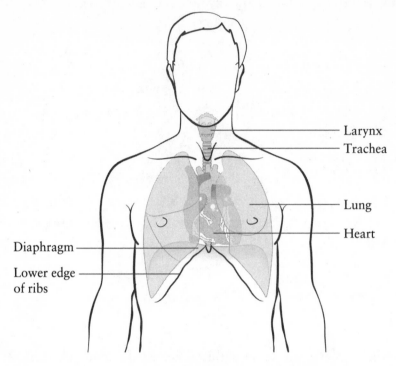

Larynx

Trachea

Lung

Heart

Diaphragm

Lower edge
of ribs

Heart and Body

What was so fascinating about heart surgery was the movement, like watching a pianist's hands or a dancer's feet. The heart beats more than sixty times per minute to pump 5 liters of blood. This adds up to 3,600 beats an hour and 80,000 in twenty-four hours. It beats 31.5 million times in a year and 2.5 billion times in eighty years. The left and right sides of the heart circulate more than 6,000 liters of blood daily to the body and lungs. An incredible workload that requires a tremendous amount of energy. And when the heart fails, there are dire consequences.

Every cell in the body needs "life blood" and oxygen. Switch this off and the tissues die at different rates. Brain first, bone last. It depends upon how much oxygen each cell needs. When the heart stops, the brain and nervous system are damaged in less than five minutes. Brain death ensues.

It was the chance to potentially save these hearts (and minds) that compelled me to the British "surgical theater," the operating room (OR).

There I found that every heart is different. Some are fat, some are lean. Some are thick, some are thin. Some are fast, some are slow. Most that I worked with were desperately sick. Twelve thousand of them, all causing misery. Crushing chest pain, interminable fatigue, terrifying breathlessness.

This book tells the stories of those hearts, and of the attempts my team and I made to save their owners. Replacing sick pumps with machines or even a dead person's heart. It's a glimpse at the edges of mortality where we operate—where breath becomes life.

one The Ether Dome

For this relief much thanks; 'tis bitter cold.
And I am sick at heart.

—*Hamlet*

THE FINEST OF MARGINS SEPARATES LIFE FROM DEATH, triumph from despair, hope from extinction. A few more dead muscle cells, a fraction more lactic acid in the blood, a little extra swelling of the brain. The Grim Reaper perches on every surgeon's shoulder. Death is always definitive. No second chances.

November 1966. I was age eighteen, a week into my first term as a student at the Charing Cross Hospital Medical School in the center of London. Having been underwhelmed with a slimy piece of lifeless muscle on the dissection table, I was impatient to see a vibrant, beating heart. I learned from a hall porter at the school that heart surgery was done across the road in the hospital on Wednesdays. Look for the Ether Dome, he told me, an antiquated leaden glass dome above the operating theater in the old Charing Cross Hospital. Find the green door on the top floor under the eaves where nobody goes. But don't get caught. Pre-clinical students were not allowed up there.

It was late in the afternoon and already dark. Drizzle was falling on the Strand. I set out to find this hidden viewing spot. Not since my entrance interview had I entered the hallowed portals of the hospital itself. We students had to earn that privilege by passing exams in anatomy, physiology, and biochemistry. So I walked quickly by the Grecian portico of the main entrance. I sneaked in through the Casualty (or Emergency) Department, under the blue light, and found an elevator—a rickety old cage used to take equipment and bodies from the wards to the basement. Inconspicuous enough.

I worried that I would be too late, that the operation would be finished. But to my delight the green door was still unlocked. Behind it, a dark, dusty corridor. Unchanged for one hundred years or more. This was a depository for obsolete anesthetic machines and discarded surgical instruments. Ten yards away I could see the glow of the operating lights beneath the dome itself. It was an old operating theater viewing gallery respectfully separated by glass from the drama below. My hand found a handrail and I lowered myself onto one of the curved wooden benches worn smooth by the restless backsides of would-be surgeons. I found myself no more than ten feet above the operating table.

I sat quietly clutching the handrail and peered through glass hazy with condensation. As the porter had promised, it was a heart operation. The chest was still open. I shifted to find the best view and settled directly above the surgeon's head. He was famous—at least in our medical school. Tall, slim, and imposing, with long fingers. In the 1960s, heart surgery was still relatively new, and its practitioners were in short supply. Few had been properly trained in the specialty. Often they were skilled general surgeons who had visited one of the pioneering heart centers, then volunteered to start a new program at their home institution. There was a steep learning curve, the cost measured in human life.

The two surgical assistants and the scrub nurse were huddled over the gaping wound, frantically shuttling instruments between them. I squinted, trying to get a closer look. And there it was, the focus of their attention and my fascination. A beating human heart. More squirming than beating. Still attached by cannulas and tubing to the heart-lung machine. Cylindrical discs were spinning through a trough of blood bathed in oxygen. A crude roller pump squeezed the tubes and accelerated this life blood back to the body. I could only see the heart. The rest of the patient was covered by green drapes and therefore anonymous, a relief to all concerned.

The surgeon restlessly shifted his weight from boot to boot, those big white operating boots that surgeons used to wear to keep blood off their socks. On the wall behind me I spotted a box labeled "Intercom." I threw the switch. Now the drama had a sound track. I learned that they had replaced the patient's mitral valve, but the heart was struggling to separate from the bypass machine. This was the first time I had seen a beating human heart, but even to me it looked feeble. Blown up like a balloon, pulsating but not pumping. Against the din of amplified background noise, I heard the surgeon say, "Let's give it one last go. Increase the adrenaline. Ventilate, and let's try to come off."

There was silence as everyone watched the desperate organ fight for its life.

"There's air in the right coronary," the first assistant said. "Give me an air needle." He shoved the needle into the aorta. Frothy blood fizzed into the wound. The blood pressure started to improve. Sensing the window of opportunity, the surgeon turned to the perfusionist—the specialist responsible for the heart-lung machine—and said, "Come off now! This is our last chance."

"Off bypass," came the tentative reply.

The heart-lung machine was switched off. The heart was now free-standing. Left ventricle pumping blood to the body, right ventricle to the lungs. Both struggling. The anesthetist stared hopefully at the screen, watching the jagged lines indicating blood pressure and heart rate. Understanding that this was the last attempt, the surgeons silently withdrew the cannulas from the heart and sewed up the holes. All willing it to get stronger. For a while it fluttered feebly, but the pressure drifted down. There was bleeding somewhere. Not torrential but persistent. Somewhere at the back. Somewhere inaccessible.

Lifting the heart caused it to fibrillate. It was now squirming, not contracting. Wriggling like a bag of worms. Incoordinate electrical activity. Wasted energy. It took the anesthetist a while to spot this on his screen. "VF," he shouted. I would learn that it meant ventricular fibrillation. "Shock it." The surgeon already knew. He was holding the defibrillating paddles hard against the heart expectantly. "30 joules"—zap. No change. "Give it 60"—zap. This time it defibrillated but went still, stunned and devoid of electrical activity. Asystole as we call it. Blood continued to fill the chest. The surgeon poked it with a finger. The ventricles responded by contracting. He poked it again and the rhythm returned. "Too slow—give me a syringe of adrenaline." The needle was shoved unceremoniously through the right ventricle into the left. The syringe squirted in clear liquid. Then he massaged the heart with his long fingers to push the powerful stimulant into the coronary arteries.

The grateful heart muscle responded rapidly. Straight out of the textbook, the heart rate accelerated, then the blood pressure soared. The barometer rose. Up and up, dangerously testing the stitches. Then, as if in slow motion, the cannula site in the aorta gave way. Whoosh. The crimson fountain hit the operating lights, sprayed the surgeons, soaked the green drapes. Someone murmured, "Oh shit." An understatement. The battle was lost.

Before a finger could plug the hole, the heart was empty. Rivulets of blood streamed across the white marble floor and dripped from the lights overhead. Rubber soles stuck to it. The anesthetist frantically squeezed bags of blood into the veins, but to no avail. Life ebbed away. As the injected slug of adrenaline wore off, the turgid heart simply blew up like a balloon and stopped. Stopped for good.

The surgeons stood silent. Despairing as they did week after week. Now the senior surgeon walked out of my view. The anesthetist turned off the ventilator and waited for the electrocardiogram (ECG) to flatline. He removed the tube from the patient's windpipe. Then he left. The brain was already dead.

Just yards away, mist descended on the Strand. Commuters rushed into Charing Cross Station to avoid the rain. Late lunches were finishing at Simpson's and Rules. Cocktails were shaken in the Waldorf and the Savoy. That was life, this was death. A lonely death on the operating table. No more pain, no more breathlessness, no more anything.

The perfusionist wheeled out his machine. It would take hours to disassemble, clean, restore, and sterilize for the next patient. Only the scrub nurse lingered. Then she was joined by the anesthetic nurse who had comforted the patient in the anteroom. They took off their masks and stared at the body. Unconcerned by the sticky blood that covered every surface. Unconcerned by the chest still splinted open. The anesthetic nurse searched for the patient's hand beneath the drapes and held it. The scrub nurse pulled away the blood-soaked covering from the face and stroked it. I could see it was a young woman.

They were oblivious to the fact that I was watching from above. No one had seen me there. I gingerly shifted along the bench to look at the patient's face. The eyes were wide open, staring into the dome. She was ashen white but still beautiful. Fine cheekbones and jet-black hair.

Like the nurses, I couldn't leave. I needed to know what happened next. They peeled back the bloodied drapes from her naked body. My brain was screaming for them to take out that hideous metal retractor cranking open her breastbone. Let her heart go back where it belongs. They did. The ribs recoiled and the poor lifeless organ was covered again. It lay flat, empty and defeated in its own space, now just a fearsome deep gash separated her tender, swollen breasts.

The intercom was still switched on. The nurses started to talk. "What will happen to her baby?"

"Adopted, I guess. She wasn't married. Her parents were killed in the Blitz."

"Where did she live?"

"Whitechapel. I think maybe the London don't do heart surgery yet. She got really sick during the pregnancy. Rheumatic fever. She nearly died during the delivery. Might have been for the best."

"Where is the baby now?"

"On the ward, I think. Matron will have to deal with it."

This was so matter of fact. A young woman had died. Her baby left without a relative in the world. No more love. No more warmth. Gone amid that tangled blood-soaked technology in the operating theater. This was what I aspired to. Was I ready?

Two student nurses came to wash the body. I recognized them from the Friday night freshers dance. They were respectful public schoolgirls. They brought a bucket of soapy water with sponges and set about scrubbing the body. They removed all of the tubing but were visibly upset by the wound and what lay beneath. Blood kept dripping out of it. "What did she have done?" said the girl I had danced with. "Heart operation, obviously," came the reply. "Valve replacement, I guess. Poor kid. She's only our age. Bet her mum's upset." They covered the wound with gauze and tape to soak up the fluid.

The scrub nurse returned and called back the surgical resident to close over the wound before the move to the mortuary. All deaths on the operating table are referred to the coroner for autopsy. She would be sliced open again, so there was no point in closing the breastbone or bringing together the different layers of the chest wall. The resident took a big needle and stitched the opening temporarily with thick braid. But the wound edges still gaped and oozed serum.

It was now 6:30 p.m. I was supposed to be in the pub down the road getting pissed with the rugby team. But something compelled me to stay. I was attached to this empty shell. This skinny corpse I had never met but now felt I knew intimately. I had been with her at the single-most-important event of her life.

The three nurses manhandled her into a starched white shroud with a ruff around the neck. Tied at the back. They then secured her ankles with tape. She was beginning to stiffen with rigor mortis. The students had done their job with kindness and respect. I knew that I would meet them again. Maybe ask them how they felt.

There were just the two of us left. The corpse and me. The operating lights still shone on her face. She was staring straight up. Why hadn't they closed her eyes like they did in the movies? I could see through those dilated pupils to the pain etched on her brain. From the fragments of conversation and with a little medical knowledge, I could evoke her life story. She was in her twenties. Born in the East End. She could only have been a small child when her parents were killed in the bombing. As a child she carries the scars of those sights and sounds. The fear of being alone as her world disintegrates. Brought up in poverty, she develops rheumatic fever. A simple sore throat that triggers a devastating inflammatory process. Rheumatic fever was common in areas of deprivation and overcrowding. Perhaps she had painful swollen joints for a few weeks. What she didn't know was that the same process was happening in her heart valves. There was no diagnostic test in those days.

She develops chronic rheumatic heart disease and is known as a sickly child. Perhaps she develops rheumatic chorea. Involuntary jerky movements, unsteady gait, and emotional turmoil. She gets pregnant. Perhaps that's an occupational hazard. This makes things worse. Her wounded heart must work that much harder. She becomes breathless and swollen but makes it through to term. Maybe the London Hospital delivers her safely but recognizes heart failure. A murmur. A leaking mitral valve. They prescribe the heart drug Digoxin, but she doesn't take it. Soon she is too tired and breathless to look after the baby. She cannot lie flat. With worsening heart failure, her outlook is grim. They send her to the city to see a surgeon. A real gentleman in a morning suit, pinstripe trousers. He is kind and sympathetic. He says only surgery on her mitral valve can help. But it didn't. It terminated her brief, hard life and left another orphan in the East End.

When the porters came, the operating lights were switched off. The mortuary trolley, a tin coffin on wheels, was drawn up alongside the operating table. By now her limbs were rigid. The body was unceremoniously dragged into this human sardine can. Her head bounced with a sickening thud, but nothing could hurt her anymore. I was relieved to lose eye contact. A green woolen blanket was folded over the top of the box to make it resemble an ordinary trolley. Then away they went to put her in the fridge. Her baby would never see her again, would never have a mother again. Welcome to cardiac surgery.

I sat there, arms on the rail, chin on my hands, staring at the black rubber surface of the empty operating table. Staring down from the Ether Dome as generations had before me. The Ether Dome was a gladiatorial arena. People came here to look down on a spectacle of life or death. Perhaps if others had witnessed it alongside me, it might have seemed less brutal. Someone to share the shock of this poor girl's death, the misery for her child.

Auxiliary nurses appeared, with mops and buckets. There to wipe away the last traces. Her blood now dry on the floor. Bloody footprints heading toward the door. Blood on the anesthetic machine, blood on the operating lights. Blood everywhere now meticulously cleaned away. A slip of a girl reaching up to clean the operating light saw me in the dome. My pale face and staring eyes against the gloom. It frightened her. My cue to leave. But one spot of dried blood remained on top of the light where no one could see. Adherent and black. It said, part of me is still here. Remember me. The green door closed behind me and I walked away. Down the shuddering lift where her body had been taken to lie in a cold fridge in the mortuary.

Notices of autopsies were posted on a board in the entrance hall of the medical school. Usually the patients were elderly. Young ones were either drug addicts, road-traffic accidents, suicides from the underground system, or cardiac surgery patients. Friday morning, I found her on the list. She was called Beth. Not Elizabeth, just Beth. She was twenty-six years old. It had to be her.

On the day of the autopsy the bodies were brought from the hospital mortuary in the basement. They were dragged under the road to the medical school in a tin box on rails by a pulley system. Then up the lift to the autopsy room. Should I go? Should I watch her insides and brain be cut out? Watch her dead heart carved into slices? Tell them how she really died, in a crimson fountain?

I couldn't do it.

Beth taught me an important lesson that day in the Ether Dome. Never get involved. Walk away as her surgeons did. Try again tomorrow. Sir Russell Brock, the most renowned British heart surgeon of the era, was known for his bluntness about losing patients. At the Royal Brompton Hospital, he used to say, "I have three patients on my operating list today—I wonder which one will survive." This may seem insensitive, even callous, but to dwell on death was a dreadful mistake. It was then. It still is now. We must learn from failure and try to do better the next time.

To indulge in sorrow or regret brings unsustainable misery. I grappled with this later in my career, when my interests veered toward the sharp end. Specializing in heart surgery for complex congenital anomalies in babies and young children, I daily walked the tightrope between the beginning and the end of life. Some patients came toddling happily into the hospital, teddy bear in one hand, mummy holding the other. Blue lips, little chest heaving, blood as thick as honey. They had never known a different life. I strived to provide that for them. To make them pink and energetic. In good faith, yet sometimes without success. What could I do? Sit with the weeping parents in a dark mortuary, holding a cold, lifeless hand? Blaming myself for taking that risk? All heart surgery is a risk. Those of us who do it don't look back. We move on to the next. Always expecting the outcome to be better. Never doubting it.

two   Humble Beginnings

Courage is doing what you're afraid to do.
There can be no courage unless you're scared.

—Eddie V. Rickenbacker

JULY 27, 1948. IT WAS THE POSTWAR BABY BOOM. AT 6:30 IN the morning, I arrived at the Maternity Department of Scunthorpe War Memorial Hospital, wailing from the depths of my newly expanded lungs.

My mother brought me safely back from the carnage of the delivery suite. Bleeding and exhausted after a long and painful labor, but happy to finally meet her first child. A pink, robust son, star sign Leo.

My mother was an intelligent woman, caring and gentle, well-liked. During the war she had managed a small business-district bank, and even with other assistants freely available, the old folks would still queue to tell her their troubles. My father joined the Royal Air Force at sixteen to fight the Germans. After the war, he got a job in the local co-op's grocery department and worked hard to improve our circumstances. Scunthorpe was a deprived and grimy steel town some two hundred miles north of London. The poor man's Pittsburgh.

Life wasn't easy. We were church-mouse poor in a grimy public-housing complex. House number thirteen. No pictures allowed on the walls in case the plaster crumbled. We had a corrugated tin air-raid shelter in the backyard that housed geese and chickens—and the outside toilet.

My maternal grandparents lived directly across the street. Grandmother was kindly and protective of me, but frail. Grandfather worked in the steel rolling mills but during the war had been the local air-raid warden. On payday I would accompany him to the steelworks to collect his wages. I was intrigued by the spectacle of white-hot molten metal pouring into ingots. Sweaty, bare-chested men in flat caps stoked the furnaces, steam trains belched fire, clanking up and down between the rolling mills and the slag heaps, sparks flying everywhere.

Grandfather patiently taught me to draw and paint. He would sit over me, puffing away on his favorite Woodbines as I painted red night skies over the chimneys, street lamps, and railway trains. There were no golden sunsets in Scunthorpe, but when the blast furnaces opened at night, the whole sky lit up. Grandfather smoked twenty cigarettes a day and spent his whole life working in smoke. It wasn't the best recipe for a long and healthy life, but no one knew that then.

In 1955, we got our first television set. A ten-inch-square box, with a grainy black-and-white picture and just one channel, the BBC. Television dramatically increased my awareness of the outside world. That year two Cambridge scientists, James Watson and Francis Crick, described the molecular structure of DNA. In Oxford, the physician Richard Doll linked smoking with lung cancer. Then came exciting news that would shape the rest of my life. Surgeons in America had closed a hole in the heart with a new machine. They called it the heart-lung machine because it took over the functions of both.

The program was called *Your Life in Their Hands*. The doctors on the television wore long white coats down to the floor. The nurses had fine starched uniforms, white caps, and rarely spoke. The patients sat stiffly at attention with their bedsheets folded back. Politely grateful for our new National Health Service (NHS).

The show described heart operations in the United States and revealed that surgeons at the Hammersmith Hospital in London would attempt one soon. They, too, would close holes in the heart. This seven-year-old street kid was captivated. Right then I decided that I would be a heart surgeon.

At age ten I passed the tests for entry to the local grammar school. By now I was focused on my goal of becoming one of those white-coated doctors. As one of the "promising" set, I was forced to work hard. I loved art, but I had to stop those classes in favor of academic subjects. But one thing was clear: I was good with my hands. My fingertips connected with my brain.

One afternoon after school, I was out walking with Grandfather and Whisky, his Highland terrier, on the outskirts of town when he stopped short on a hill and began clutching the collar of his shirt. His head bowed and his skin drained of color. Sweating and breathless, he sank to the ground. He couldn't speak. I could see the fear in his eyes. I wanted to run and fetch the doctor, but Grandfather wouldn't let me. He couldn't risk being off work, even at the age of fifty-eight. I held his head until the pain abated. It lasted thirty minutes, and once he'd recovered we slowly made for home.

My grandfather's ill health wasn't news to my mother. She told me that he had been getting a lot of "indigestion" while cycling to work. Reluctantly, he agreed to get off the bike, but it didn't do much good. The episodes became more frequent, even at rest, and especially when he would climb the stairs, gasping for breath. Cold was bad for his chest, so the old iron bed was brought down and put in front of the fire, the commode brought inside to save a journey outdoors.

His ankles and calves became so swollen with fluid that he needed bigger shoes. It was a gargantuan effort even to tie his shoelaces. He didn't get out much. Mostly, he moved from the bed to a chair in front of the fire. I would sit and draw for him to take his mind off his distressing symptoms.

One wet afternoon in November, the day before President Kennedy was assassinated in Dallas, I came home from school to find a black Austin Healy outside my grandparents' house. It was the doctor's car. I knew instinctively what that meant. I stared through condensation on the front window, but the curtains were drawn. I went around the back of the house and walked in quietly through the kitchen door. I could hear sobbing. My heart sank.

The living room door was ajar and the room was dimly lit. I peered in. The doctor stood by the bed with a syringe in his hand. My mother and grandmother were clasped together at the end of the bed. Grandfather was ashen gray with a heaving chest. His head was tipped back and frothy pink fluid dripped from his blue lips and purple nose. He coughed agonally, spraying bloody foam over the sheets. Then his head fell to his shoulder, wide eyes staring at the wall, fixed on the placard that said "Bless this house." The doctor felt for a pulse at the wrist, then whispered, "He's gone." A sense of peace and relief descended on the room. His suffering was at an end.

The certificate would say: "Death from heart failure." I slipped out unnoticed to sit with the chickens in the air-raid shelter and quietly disintegrated. Now I understood what that glib phrase "heart failure" really meant and why those surgeons in America strived to make a difference. Unbeknownst to me at the time, this tragic event was destined to shape my whole future.

Soon afterward, my grandmother was diagnosed with thyroid cancer. It started to close off her windpipe. *Stridor* is the medical term to describe the sound of strangulation as the ribs and diaphragm struggle to force air through the narrowed airway. She went to the city of Lincoln, forty miles away, for radiotherapy, but it burned the skin and made swallowing more difficult. We were given hope of relief by a surgical tracheostomy. But when the surgeon attempted the procedure, he couldn't position the hole low enough in the windpipe, below the narrowing. Our hopes were dashed. My grandmother, like her husband, was doomed to suffer until she died. It would have been better if they had allowed her to go under the anesthetic. Every evening, I sat with her after school, doing what I could to make her comfortable. Soon opiate drugs and carbon-dioxide narcosis clouded her consciousness. One night she slipped away with a large brain hemorrhage. At sixty-three, she had been the longest lived of my grandparents.

At sixteen, I took jobs over the school holidays to boost our income. I worked for the steelworks for a while, but after I caused a collision between my dumper truck and a diesel train hauling molten iron, the works dispensed with my services. Perhaps for the best, as I almost died that day! Then, to my excitement, I spotted a temporary portering job at the local hospital and negotiated the role of operating theater porter. I quickly learned how to please the various constituents: The patients, fasted, fearful, and lacking dignity in their hospital gowns, needed kindness, reassurance, and handling with respect. Junior nurses were friendly and fun. The nursing sisters were self-important, bossy, and businesslike. Even at sixteen, I knew what they needed. The anesthetists didn't want to be kept waiting. The surgeons were arrogant and ignored me—at first.

One of my jobs was to help transfer the bodies of the anesthetized patients from the trolley to the operating table. As an artist, I was intrigued by anatomy. Knowing what surgery was planned from the operating list, I began to help by adjusting the overhead lights, focusing them on the site of the incision. Gradually the surgeons began to take notice of my efforts. Some inquired about my interest. I told them that I was determined to be a heart surgeon one day. Soon enough, I was allowed to watch the surgeries.

Working nights was fascinating because of the emergencies. Horrific injuries from the works. Broken bones, dead guts, and bleeding aneurysms were all more frequent after dark. Most of the aneurysm cases died. The nurses cleaned the corpses and put on the shrouds, then I hauled them from the operating table onto the tin mortuary trolley. They always landed with a dull thud. Then I'd wheel them to the mortuary and stack the bodies in the cold store. You get used to it.

Inevitably, my first mortuary visit was in the dead of night. The windowless gray brick building was set apart from the main hospital. I was terrified of what I would find there. I turned the key in the heavy wooden door that led directly into the autopsy room. I couldn't find the light switch, but I had a flashlight. The beam danced around the green-tiled walls, reflected from white marble slabs and glistening sharp instruments, as I plucked up the courage to go in. It smelled of death. Or what I expected death to smell like. Stacks of square metal doors stretched from floor to ceiling—the cold store. I needed to find a fridge but wasn't sure which ones were empty. Eventually, the torch beam found a light switch and I turned on the overhead fluorescents. It didn't make me feel any better.

Some doors had a piece of cardboard with a name on it. I figured that they must be occupied. So I turned the handle on an unmarked fridge. There I found a white linen sheet covering a naked old woman. An anonymous corpse. Damn. Try again on the second tier. This time lucky. I pulled out the sliding tin tray and pushed the creaking mechanical hoist toward my corpse. How to make this thing work without dropping the body on the floor? Straps, crank handles, and manhandling. I got on with it and slid the tray back into the fridge. Success. But as I bolted the door in relief came the realization that my corpse was anonymous, too. No cardboard label. I had forgotten to ask the dead patient's name. So I left a cryptic note: "Occupied—will bring details in the morning."

The mortuary door was still wide open, as I was scared of being shut in there alone. I sped out, pushing the squeaking mortuary trolley back to the main hospital, ready for the next body. I wondered how pathologists could spend half of their career in that environment, carving entrails from the dead on marble slabs.

Yet curiosity won out over my initial distaste. Eventually, I charmed an older female pathologist into letting me watch the autopsies. Even after witnessing some disfiguring operations and terrible trauma cases, this took some getting used to. Young and old sliced open from throat to pubis. Eviscerated. Scalp incised from ear to ear and peeled forward over the face like an orange. The cranium sawed open like taking the top off a boiled egg. The whole human brain in front of me. How does this soft gray convoluted mass govern our whole lives? I pondered. And how could surgeons possibly operate on this wobbly jelly?

I learned so much in that dingy, bleak autopsy room. The complexity of human anatomy, the psychology of detachment. There was no room for sentiment in pathology. An ounce of compassion maybe, but affinity with the cadaver? No. Forget the heart as the source of love and devotion. Or the brain as the seat of the soul. Whoever these cadavers used to be, the pathologists had to get on and slice them up. Soon I could identify a coronary thrombosis, a myocardial infarction, a rheumatic heart valve, or a dissected aorta. Or cancer spread to the liver or lungs. The common stuff. I learned how charred or decomposed bodies smelled. (Vicks VapoRub stuffed up the nostrils spared the olfactory nerves.)

Yet it was difficult not to feel sad for the young who came through. Babies, children, and teenagers with cancer or deformed hearts. Those whose lives were destined, whether by biology or accident, to be short and miserable. Suicides. When I mentioned this, I was told to "get over it if you want to be a surgeon." And that it would all be easier when I could drink. I sensed that alcohol was high on the list of surgeons' recreational activities. It became more obvious when they were called in at night. But who was I to judge?

At the same time, I began to wonder whether I could actually get into medical school. I was no great academic. I struggled with math and physics, the subjects that, for me, were the real barometer of intelligence. Yet I excelled in biology and could get by with chemistry. In the end I passed my exams. Stuff I would never need like Latin and French literature. Additional math and religious studies. All of that was a function of effort, not intelligence. But hard work was my route out of those grimy backstreets. My ticket to a different life. And the time spent in the hospital had made me worldly. I had never left Scunthorpe, but I knew about life and death.

I started to search for a way to enter medical school, continuing to work at the hospital during every school holiday. In my job, I eventually climbed my way up to the position of "Operating Department assistant." An expert in cleaning up blood, vomit, bone dust, and shit. Humble beginnings.

I was shocked when I was called for an interview at a magnificent Cambridge college. Someone must have put in a good word, though I never learned who. The streets bustled with lively young students in their gowns. Chatting loudly with upper-crust accents, they seemed much smarter than me. Erudite, bespectacled professors cycled through cobbled streets in their mortarboards, off to college dinners for wine and port. My mind flashed back to the grimy steelworkers silently making their way home in flat caps and mufflers. For bread and potatoes, maybe a glass of stout. My spirits started to sink. I didn't belong here.

The interview was conducted by two distinguished fellows in an oak-paneled study overlooking the main college quadrangle. We sat in well-worn leather armchairs. It was meant to be a relaxed atmosphere. Nothing was said about my background. The promised question, "Why do you want to study medicine?" never came. Wasted interview practice. I was asked why the Americans had invaded Vietnam. Had I heard of any tropical disease their soldiers might be exposed to? I didn't know whether there was malaria in Vietnam so I said "syphilis." That broke the ice. I suggested that this might be less of a health problem than napalm and bullets. Next. Winston Churchill had just died. Did I think that smoking cigars may have contributed to his demise? Smoking was one of the key words I had been waiting for. My mouth fired off in automatic mode: cancer, bronchitis, coronary artery disease, myocardial infarction, heart failure. How they looked in the autopsy room. Had I seen an autopsy? Many. (And cleared up the brains, guts, and bodily fluids afterward.) "Thank you. We'll let you know in a few weeks' time." With that, I walked away through the ancient, cobbled streets, feeling dejected. For me, Cambridge was a different world.

Next I was called down to the Charing Cross Hospital on the Strand. Located between Trafalgar Square and Covent Garden Market, the old hospital was built to serve the poor of Central London and had a distinguished war history. The interview was held in the hospital boardroom. A kindly matron received the candidates with tea and cakes. Although I arrived early, I was always last alphabetically. I twiddled my thumbs anxiously to while away what seemed like hours, making polite conversation with the matron about what had happened to the hospital during the war.

The distinguished Harley Street surgeon and chief interviewer wore a morning suit. Across the other side of the boardroom table was the famously irascible Scots professor of anatomy. The character upon whom the *Doctor in the House* television series was first based. I sat straight-backed at attention on the upright wooden chair. No slouching here. First question: What did I know about the hospital? Thank you, God. Or Matron. Next I was asked about my cricketing record and whether I could play rugby. That was all. The interview was over, the last of the day. They were tired and had had enough. They would let me know.

This time I wandered out into Covent Garden. Past the colorful market stalls and bustling taverns. All life was there. Tramps, tarts, buskers, and bankers. The Charing Cross Hospital clientele. Black cabs and scarlet London buses streamed down the Strand. Meandering between the crowds and the traffic, I came to the grand entrance of the Savoy Hotel. I wondered whether I should dare to go in. I surely looked smart enough in my interview suit and Brylcreemed hair. Before I'd made up my mind, the immaculate doorman pushed the swing doors open and ushered me through. "Welcome, sir." The seal of approval. I strode purposefully through the atrium, past the Savoy Grill, hesitating only to scrutinize the menu in its gilt frame. The prices! I kept walking. A sign pointed to the "American Bar." The hall was lined with signed cartoons, photographs, and paintings of the West End stars. At 5:00 p.m. there was no queue. Perched on a high stool, I furtively devoured free canapés and perused the cocktail menu. Devoid of insight, I was pushed to make a decision. "Singapore Sling, please." My first alcoholic drink. Like flipping a switch, my life had changed. From Scunthorpe to the Savoy.

Within the week a letter arrived from Charing Cross Hospital Medical School. Opening it surrounded by my anxious parents felt like defusing a bomb. Relief and excitement. They had offered me a place. The conditions: pass the biology, chemistry, and physics exams, no grades specified.

A small medical school, Charing Cross accepted only fifty students each year. I would be following in the footsteps of such distinguished alumni as Thomas Huxley, the zoologist, and David Livingstone, the explorer.

I would be the first in my family to go to university. The first doctor. And, I hoped, the first heart surgeon.

three Lord Brock's Boots

> He has been a doctor a year now and has had two patients.
> No, three. I attended their funerals.
>
> —Mark Twain

THE BEST WAY TO PREPARE FOR THE EXAMS TO BECOME A fellow of the Royal College of Surgeons was to work as an anatomy demonstrator in the dissection room of the medical school. That meant teaching anatomy to the new students in minute detail and helping them to dismantle their cadaver, layer by layer. Skin, fat, muscle, sinew, and then organs. Greasy embalmed corpses on a tin trolley. Six new and impressionable students to each. They all marched in with starched white coats and brand-new dissection kits. Scalpel, scissors, forceps, and hooks in a linen roll. Green as grass. I recognized the eager gleam in their eyes. Over the duration of the course, I moved from group to group to maintain their momentum. A few couldn't hack it. To spend untold hours picking away at a corpse was not part of their medical dream. I tried to put this in perspective for them, offer practical advice. Wear strong perfume. Don't skip breakfast. Think about something else: sports, shopping, sex. Learn enough to pass the tests. But don't let the stiffs drive you out. It worked with some. Others had nightmares. Their dissected corpse visited them at night.

For my first surgery exam, I had to master anatomy, physiology, and pathology. Nothing to do with being able to operate. There were intensive review courses in London meant to hammer home the facts, taught by past examiners who presented the information in the way that the college wanted it. Pay up and pass was the message. Yet two-thirds of candidates failed at every exam, including me on my first attempt.

In the midst of this academic monotony, the Royal Brompton Hospital advertised for "Resident Surgical Officers." Fellowship of the College of Surgeons was "desirable but not obligatory." After eight years of medical school and a residency, I had only just passed the first part of my surgical schooling. It would be a minimum of three years before I could sit the final exam. Could I aspire to the job? Nothing lost by trying, I thought.

Despite the odds, I succeeded in securing the post, and I started a few weeks later. I was allocated to work for Mr. Mattias Paneth, an imposing six-foot, six-inch German, and Mr. Christopher Lincoln, the newly appointed children's heart surgeon of similarly towering height. They were two very different personalities, yet both intimidating in their own way, at least at first. In my massively busy junior-resident jobs at Charing Cross, I learned that the only way to keep up was to write everything down. Record every order or request as it was verbalized. To forget was to be in deep shit. So I carried a clipboard. This was a source of great amusement to Mr. Paneth, who took to repeating, "Did you get that Westaby? Did you get that Westaby?"

My surgical logbook opened in spectacular fashion. The Paneth team had a case scheduled after the outpatient clinic. An elderly lady from Wales for mitral-valve replacement. The boss invited me to go and start while he saw a few more private patients. I proudly changed into the blue scrubs. Not only that, I had found a pair of white-rubber surgeon's boots in an open locker. They were well worn and dirty. I could have had new clogs but coveted these discarded second-hand boots. Why? Because down the strip at the back was written "Brock." I was about to inherit Lord Brock's boots. By now, Baron Brock of Wimbledon was seventy and had stopped operating. Paneth alluded to him as having "perpetual disappointment at the unattainability of universal perfection." President of the Royal College of Surgeons when I was at medical school, he had stayed on as director of the Department of Surgical Sciences. Now I would follow in his footsteps, literally. I strode out of the surgeons' changing room and into the operating theater to introduce myself.

The diminutive elderly lady was on the operating table, fully anesthetized. The vastly experienced scrub sister had already prepared her with antiseptic iodine solution and covered the naked body in faded green linen drapes. Now she was impatiently tapping her theater clogs on the marble floor. The long-suffering anesthetist, Dr. English, and the chief perfusionist were playing chess by the anesthetic machine. I sensed that they had been waiting for some time. I pulled on my face mask and quickly scrubbed up, relishing this first opportunity to showcase my skills.

I carefully located the landmarks. The sternal notch at the base of the neck and the tongue of cartilage at the lower end of the breastbone. The scalpel incision, a perfectly straight line cut from top to bottom, would join the two. She was thin and emaciated with heart failure. There was little fat between skin and bone to cleave with the electrocautery. At this point there was no sign of another assistant, but I pressed on regardless, seeking to impress the nurses.

I took the oscillating bone saw and tested it. Buzzzz. That was fierce enough. So I bravely started to run it up the bone toward the neck. Then, disaster. After the light spattering of bloody bone marrow, a sudden gush of dark-red blood poured from the middle of the incision. Shit! Instantly I started to sweat. Sister knew the score. She swiftly moved around to the assistant's position. I grabbed the sucker, but Sister was giving the orders. "Press hard on the bleeding." Dr. English belatedly looked up from the chessboard, unfazed by the frenetic activity. "Get me a unit of blood," he calmly told the anesthetic nurse. "Then give Mr. Paneth a call in Outpatients."

I knew what the problem was. The saw had lacerated the right ventricle. But how? There should have been a tissue space behind the sternum and fluid in the sac around the heart. Sister was reading my mind. Something she would do many times in the next six months. "You do know that this is a reoperation." A statement that was really a question. "No, absolutely not," came my response. "Where's the bloody scar?"

"It was a closed mitral valvotomy. The scar's around the side of the chest. You can just see it under her breast. Didn't Mr. Paneth tell you it was a re-do?"

I decided to keep my mouth shut. It was time for action, not recrimination.

In reoperations, the heart and surrounding tissues are stuck together by inflammatory adhesions. There is no space between the heart and the fibrous sac around it. In this case the right ventricle had stuck to the underside of the breastbone. Everything was matted together. Worse still, the right ventricle was dilated because the pressure in the pulmonary artery was high. The pressure in the pulmonary artery was high because the rheumatic mitral valve was tightly narrowed. We were there to replace the diseased valve, but I had botched it right from the start.

Pressing hadn't controlled the bleeding. Blood still poured through the bone, and the sternum wasn't completely open yet. The blood pressure began to sag. She was a small lady with not much blood to lose. Dr. English started to transfuse donor blood. But it was like pouring water into a drainpipe. In one end, straight

out the other. I was the surgeon. It was my job to stop the hemorrhage, and for that I needed to see the hole.

My own perspiration dripped into the wound and trickled down
my legs into Lord Brock's boots. The patient's blood flowed off the
drapes onto the faded white rubber. By now one of the circulating
nurses had scrubbed up and joined us at the operating table. I lifted
the saw again and asked Sister to move her hands. Through a deluge
of blood I ran the saw through the remaining intact bone, the thick
part of the sternum, below the neck. Then we pressed on the bleeding again while more transfusion restored some blood pressure. As
pressure drops, the rate of bleeding slows. This gave me the window
of opportunity to dissect the heart away from the back of the breastbone, sufficient time to insert the metal sternal retractor and wedge
open the chest. Now I could see the lacerated right ventricle spilling
its contents into the wound. When everything is stuck together like
this, spreading the bone edges can tear the heart muscle wide open.
Irretrievably so. I had been lucky. Her heart was still in one piece.
Just about.

By now my own pulse was galloping. I could see that the problem was a ragged slit 5 centimeters long in the free wall of the right
ventricle, comfortably distant from the main coronary arteries. Instinctively, Sister put her fist directly on it as I wound the retractor
open. At last this stemmed the bleeding, and we were able to bring
the blood pressure back up. The backup scrub nurse divided the
long plastic tubes to the heart-lung machine so that we could use
it when ready. As yet not enough of the heart had been exposed
for that. First I needed to stitch up the bloody hole. As a surgical
houseman, I had stitched skin, blood vessels, and guts. Never a heart.
Sister told me what stitch to use. And to be careful: "Don't tie the
knots too tight or the stitches will cut through the muscle." And to
stitch like sewing the hem of a dress. Continuous thread with full-
thickness bites, not time-consuming individual stitches, which are
slow to knot. A continuous stitch was quicker and would provide

a better seal. "Get started and you might finish before Paneth gets here and chews your head off."

The difficult part was to stitch accurately as blood poured out of the ventricle with every beat—and with gloves dripping with blood on the outside and sweat on the inside. Dr. English helped with that. He said "use the fibrillator—stop it beating for a couple of minutes." The fibrillator is an electrical device that causes what we normally never want to see: ventricular fibrillation, that unsettling quivering. That also means no blood flow to the brain at normal body temperature. In four minutes, brain damage begins.

English was reassuring. "Just defibrillate it after two minutes. If you haven't closed it by then we can wait a couple of minutes, then fibrillate again." I felt like a puppet with the experienced players pulling the strings. Fine by me. I put the fibrillating electrodes on the surface of what muscle I could see. English threw the switch. The heart stopped beating, started quivering, and I began to sew at top speed. Just as Mr. Paneth appeared at the operating theater door. He could see ventricular fibrillation on the monitor and feared the worst. But I didn't look up. I just kept on stitching. When Dr. English announced the two-minute cutoff, I had almost finished bringing the muscle edges together. I carried on to three minutes. The hole was closed. Just the knot to tie.

I put the defibrillating paddles as close to the heart as possible and said, "Defibrillate." Nothing happened. The leads to the paddles hadn't been plugged into the machine. Minor detail. Seconds ticked by. Then came the "zap" I had been waiting for. The heart briefly stood still, then fibrillated again. Paneth strode across from the door in his suit and outdoor shoes. No hat, no mask. He looked over the drapes at the quivering muscle and said the obvious. "More joules." Another zap. The heart defibrillated and started to beat vigorously. Paneth grinned, then asked, "Anything you would like to tell me, Westaby? The mitral valve isn't in the right ventricle, you know. I thought you were bright." He winked at Sister and announced that he was going for tea. Meanwhile not to let Westaby do anything stupid. I scraped my nerves from the ceiling and took stock. I tied that last knot. The heart seemed to be working fine, despite my assault. There was blood all down my gown, on Lord Brock's boots and in a pool on the floor. But the blood pressure was back to normal. Today's battle was won.

I looked at Sister. A pair of cool blue eyes above the mask. I reached for her blood-stained rubber glove to say "thanks for saving both of us." By the time Mr. Paneth took over, it was as if nothing had happened. Apart from jokes about the extra needlework on the front of the heart. I felt like screaming, "Why did not you tell me she was a fucking redo?" Then realized that he probably had no recollection of that, either. It had been many months since he had talked to her in the Outpatient Department. The rest of the operation went smoothly. Dr. English and the perfusionist continued their chess game. I held the sucker. Paneth cut out the deformed valve and replaced it with a "ball in cage" prosthesis. Lots of stitching.

There was no end to the day for surgical residents. That night I sat in the Intensive Care Unit (ICU) waiting for the lady to wake up. Desperately hoping that she wasn't brain-damaged. And wondering how I would have felt had she bled out on the operating theater floor. Would I have had the grit to continue? Such a fine line between hero and zero. I had survived. Now I just wanted her to wake up.

Her husband and daughter were keeping vigil by her bedside. Her husband asked whether the operation had gone well. I glibly said, "Yes. Very well. Mr. Paneth did a great job." Avoiding any suggestion that I had fucked up.

As if to order, she opened her eyes. A wave of relief flowed over me. Husband and daughter jumped to their feet, making sure that she could see them as she stared toward the ceiling, still transfixed by the breathing tube. They reached out for her hand. At that point I realized something. Heart surgery might become an everyday occurrence for me. But usually for the patient and their relatives, it is once in a lifetime. And absolutely terrifying. I reminded myself to treat them kindly.

Life became different with my new profession. Cardiac surgery was like quicksand—once in it, you were sucked deeper and deeper. It was hard to leave the hospital in case something remarkable happened while I was gone. For endless hours I sat by the cots of Mr. Lincoln's babies. Listening to the bip-bip-bip of the monitors. Watching the blood pressure sag and trying to get it up again. Hoping that blood would stop dripping into the drains.

The next debacle followed quickly. One Saturday evening before Christmas, a group of residents had met in the pub following dinner in the mess. Because there was no Casualty Department at the Brompton, emergency operations were unusual at night, particularly during the weekends. With a couple of pints of beer on board, we were alerted by the switchboard that a US Air Force jet had taken off from Iceland with a young man injured in a road-traffic accident. He had a tear in the wall of the aorta, and Mr. Paneth was coming in to operate. Big problem. Both the injury and the beer. Not the amount of alcohol—we were used to that. More the volume of urine to vacate during a four-hour operation. There was no way I could maintain concentration with a bursting bladder. And I didn't want to lose face by asking to leave, like a whimpering schoolboy with his hand up in class.

As the chief resident went off to make arrangements with the operating theaters, I pondered the possibilities. What about a urinary catheter and drainage bag? I didn't relish the idea of passing the catheter myself. Nor the discomfort of standing with the bag of urine strapped to my leg. Then it dawned on me. Lord Brock's operating theater boots. One of them would hold a couple of pints. And Paul's tubing—long, thin-walled rubber tubing that used to be used for incontinent males. Less risk of a bladder infection than if I inserted my own catheter.

I went to the wards in search of the tubing. It came in a roll that I cut to the length of my inside leg. Then off I went to the surgeons' changing room. I was eager to be already in the theater as the boss arrived. With my clipboard and white boots as usual, tubing attached with sticky tape all ready to go.

The ambulance arrived from Heathrow sooner than we had anticipated. We were opening the left side of the chest by midnight and soon encountered bleeding. Paneth was irascible, having been called out of a Christmas party. As predicted, my resident colleague became restless with bladder fullness. Shifting from foot to foot. Losing concentration. Eventually he had to excuse himself. I moved into the first-assistant position, coughing loudly to disguise the unusual squelching sound. I stayed there even after the resident returned. I had no discomfort. Unbeknownst to the others, I was slowly filling my right Wellington boot. After another twenty minutes, the resident had to go out again. By now the patient was safe, but Paneth was cross. "What's wrong with him? He's been in the pub hasn't he? He's been drinking." I said, "I really don't know, Mr. Paneth. I've been studying in the library all evening." I waited to be struck down by a thunderbolt, but it never came. The response was predictable. "Well done, Westaby. You get on and close the chest. He can assist you for a change. See you on Monday." I disposed of the evidence and accompanied the young patient back to the ICU. No one ever knew.

Now beyond sleep, I sat drinking coffee in the pediatric ICU. Talking with the nurses. Watching tiny people struggle for life in their cosy incubators for Christmas. As surgical trainees, we were all chronically sleep-deprived. There was little excitement in sleep. Sleep was something for the odd weekend off. All adrenaline junkies, we lived on a continuous high. Craving action. From bleeding patients to cardiac arrests. From operating theater to ICU. From pub to party.

Sleep deprivation is what underpins the psychopathy of the surgical mind. Immunity to stress, an ability to take risks, the loss of empathy. Bit by bit, I was being inducted into that exclusive club.

four Township Boy

Genius is 1 percent inspiration and 99 percent perspiration.

—Thomas Edison

OCTOBER 1979. I WAS CHIEF RESIDENT WITH THE THO-racic surgery service at Harefield Hospital in North London. Everyone training in heart surgery had to learn to operate on the lungs and esophagus, too. This meant working with cancer, which in those days I found deeply depressing. Too often it had already spread to other parts of the body, and for most patients the progno-sis was grim. So they were depressed, too. Moreover, there was an element of monotony about it. Should we take out half a lung or the whole lung? On the right or on the left? Remove the upper part of the gullet or the lower half? After doing each one hundred times, it wasn't very stimulating.

Every so often a more challenging case would present itself. Mario was an Italian engineer working on a restoration project in Saudi Arabia. A jovial family man, he had gone there hoping to earn enough money to buy a house, working hours on end at a large industrial complex outside of Jeddah in the searing desert heat. Then, catastrophe. Without warning, while Mario was working in an enclosed area, a huge boiler exploded, filling the atmosphere with steam. Steam under high pressure. It scalded his face and burned the lining of his windpipe and bronchial tubes. The shock almost killed him immediately.

The scalded tissues were dead. Whole sheets of necrotic membrane sloughed off from the lining of his bronchial tubes. This obstructive debris had to be removed through an old-fashioned rigid bronchoscope, a long brass tube with a light on the end, passed through the back of the throat and voice box, then down into the airways. Mario needed this done regularly to prevent asphyxiation. But pushing the bronchoscope back and forth through his larynx became more and more difficult. Soon, it became so scarred that the bronchoscope would not pass. He needed a tracheostomy—a surgical hole in the neck to allow him to breathe. Next, as his condition worsened, the dead bronchial lining was replaced with inflammatory tissue. Masses of cells started to fill the airways like calcium blocking water pipes. He couldn't breathe. The progress was relentless and downhill.

I took the call from Jeddah. The burns doctor looking after him explained the dire situation and wondered whether we had any advice. Mario was only forty-two. I suggested they airlift him to Heathrow, and we would see if anything could be done. The building company paid for the medical evacuation, and he arrived the following day. At the time, my boss was in the twilight of his career and was happy for me to take on as much as I felt confident doing. Which was everything. I had no fear. But this was an awful injury in a young man. I asked my superior whether we might take a look down his windpipe together and then try to come up with a plan.

Mario was a sorry sight. He was gasping for breath, with infected froth pouring from his tracheostomy tube, which made a dreadful, gurgling sound. His scarlet face was badly burned, with crusted dead skin peeling away. Weeping serum. Burned on the outside and burned on the inside. It was a great relief for him to be anesthetized.

As he lapsed into unconsciousness, I sucked blood-stained sticky secretions from the hole in the neck. Then attached the tubing from the ventilator to the tracheostomy tube and squeezed the black rubber bag. The lungs were difficult to inflate against the resistance of obstructing inflammatory tissue. I decided that we should attempt to pass the rigid bronchoscope by the normal route. Directly through the vocal cords and larynx, akin to sword swallowing, but down the airways, not the gullet. We needed a view of the whole windpipe and both right and left main bronchial tubes. For this the head needs to be tipped at the correct angle to visualize the vocal cords at the back of the throat. We do our best not to knock out any teeth. We used to perform this technique on conscious individuals after lung surgery. I had to vacuum the patients out because there were never enough physiotherapists on staff to do the job. It was rough at the time, but better than drowning.

I maneuvered the rigid telescope over the teeth and along the back of the tongue. Then peered down to find the snippet of cartilage known as the epiglottis, which protects the opening of the voice box during swallowing. Lift the tip with the bronchoscope and there should be the glistening white vocal cords with a vertical slit between them. That's the way in to the windpipe. I had done this hundreds of times to biopsy lung cancer. Or remove peanuts. This was not the same. The voice box was burned, the vocal cords like sausages, inflamed and angry looking. There was no way through. Mario was entirely reliant on the tracheostomy.

Standing aside, I tried to show my boss. Keeping the bronchoscope still, propped on the teeth. He grunted and shook his head. "Try pushing it harder. Nothing to lose I suspect." Taking aim again, I pushed the beak of the scope where the slit should be and shoved. The swollen vocal cords parted and the instrument crashed against the tracheostomy tube. We attached the ventilating apparatus to the side of the bronchoscope and pulled out the tube. Normally we would see the full length of the windpipe, down to where it divides into the main bronchi. Not a chance here. The airways were virtually obliterated by the proliferating cells. I eased the rigid implement onward, using the sucker to aspirate blood and detached tissue. At the same time pushing in oxygen through the bronchoscope tip, hoping to see an end to the burns. We finally encountered normal airway lining halfway down each main bronchial tube. Now the traumatized lining was oozing blood.

Mario's bright-red face was now purple and getting bluer by the minute. The boss took over. He was peering down the tube, occasionally inserting the long telescope for a better view. It was a precarious situation without an obvious solution. Everyone knows if you can't breathe, you die. Fortunately with time the bleeding died down. The airway was better with some gunk removed. We reinserted the tracheostomy tube and put the patient back on the ventilator. Both sides of the chest still moved. Both lungs were inflated. A triumph in itself, but it was doubtful there was any way forward. We both concluded that his prospects were bleak.

Two days later, Mario's left lung collapsed and we went through the same process again. It was just as bad. The tissue kept on growing. He remained fully conscious on the ventilator, and distressed. Asphyxiation is the most miserable way to die. I remembered my grandmother, strangulated by cancer of the thyroid gland, told she needed a tracheostomy only to have the procedure aborted. So she sat propped up in bed day and night, gasping for breath. I remembered trying to work out ways to help. Why wasn't it possible to put a tube farther down past the obstruction? Why couldn't tracheostomy tubes be made longer? A simple concept, but I was repeatedly told it wasn't possible.

From what I could see through the bronchoscope, the situation with Mario was nearly identical. He needed something to bypass his whole trachea and both main bronchi, or he would be dead within days. We couldn't keep opening the airways with a bronchoscope indefinitely. The Grim Reaper was winning this battle. About to swing the scythe.

Ever the optimist, I grasped for alternative solutions. Could we make a branched tube to bypass the damaged airways? The boss thought it would clog with secretions. And someone else would have done it before for cancer. Then came an afterthought. A company called Hood Laboratories in Boston, Massachusetts, was making a silicone rubber tube with a tracheostomy side limb. They called it a Montgomery T tube after its ear, nose, and throat surgeon inventor. Maybe I could talk to the company and explain the problem.

When I bronchoscoped Mario later that afternoon, I took measurements to calculate how long the tube needed to be to reach down each main bronchus. That evening, I rang Hood. The company confirmed that no one had tried such an approach but agreed to make me the bifurcated tube to fit the whole of Mario's trachea and main bronchial tubes. I emphasized that we needed it urgently. They delivered in less than one week, with no invoice, pleased to help with this unique case. Now I had to work out how to get it in.

I would need to railroad the branched end of the tube into the separate bronchi simultaneously over guidewires. But wires were too sharp and dangerous for the delicate silicone rubber. I needed something blunt and harmless. We used to dilate strictures of the gullet with gum elastic bougies, which are thin, flexible dilators. Two of the narrowest bougies would fit down the T-Y tube, and down each limb of the Y branches. I could insert the bougies through the damaged trachea and into one bronchus at a time, then railroad the tube into place over them. I drew the technique step by step and showed it to the other thoracic surgeons. The consensus was that we had nothing to lose. Without some crazy new approach, Mario was going to die.

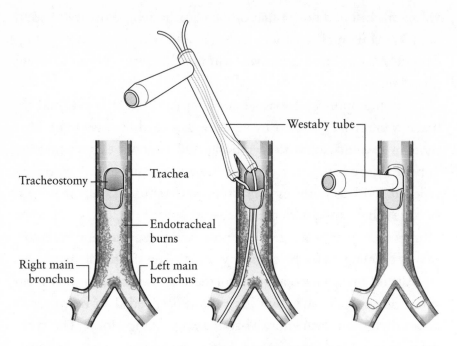

Insertion of the Westaby Tube

The following day we took him to the operating theater, removed the tracheostomy tube, and inserted the rigid bronchoscope through the burned larynx. I tried to create as little bleeding as possible. We surgically enlarged the tracheostomy hole through which the T-Y tube would be introduced. Then the bougies were inserted into the right and left main bronchi under direct vision through the scope, vigorously ventilating with 100 percent oxygen between each step. So far so good. I lubricated the silicone rubber with K-Y jelly and shoved the tube forcefully downward. The bronchial limbs spread out at the branching point until there was resistance to any further pushing. It was in. The boss took the leap of faith and withdrew the bronchoscope into the larynx.

Ever the Irishman, he exclaimed, "Crikey, look at this! You're a bloody genius, Westaby." The horribly disintegrating trachea was replaced with a clean white silicone tube. The Y limbs sat in perfect position. There was no kinking or compression, and clean healthy airways beyond.

Meanwhile, Mario was blue and hypoxic. We were all so excited that we had stopped ventilating him. Now we needed to blow in oxygen furiously. But he was easy to inflate through the wide rubber airways.

It was a revelation. Whether it would last we didn't know. Only time would tell. It depended entirely upon whether Mario was strong enough to cough secretions out through the tubes. And upon our ability to suck them out and ventilate him through the side limb. When the swelling in the larynx and vocal cords subsided, we planned to keep this closed with the rubber plug. Then he could breathe, humidify the inspired air, and speak through his own larynx, if it ever recovered. There were many unknowns, but for now Mario was safe. He could breathe. He woke up with fantastic symptomatic relief.

I should have been thrilled that the concept worked. But beyond the initial satisfaction of feeling the rubber tube fit in place, I wasn't. Despite my professional successes, I was troubled in my personal life. I had been married, with a beautiful baby daughter, Gemma, whom I didn't live with. I aspired to a career caring for children, yet I neglected my own. This was grinding away at me in the background. I compensated by operating fanatically. On everything I could lay my hands on. Always available, but with a disquieting restlessness.

Mario recovered well, though life was difficult without a voice. He could cough secretions through the tube and keep it clear, something that everyone else had regarded as impossible. And he went home to his family in Italy. Gratifyingly, Hood started to manufacture the T-Y stent and called it the "Westaby Tube." We used it often for patients whose lung cancer was threatening to occlude the lower airways. It relieved the dreadful strangulation that my grandmother was forced to endure. Why could no one have done it when she needed help? When she was so miserable.

I never knew how many "Westaby Tubes" were used, but the device stayed in Hood's product list for many years. My original drawings were published in a chest-surgery journal and served as the official guide. When I was still performing thoracic surgery, I continued to use it for complex airways problems, often on a temporary basis until radiotherapy or cancer drugs caused the tumor to shrink. It was my grandmother's legacy.

Years later I had the rare opportunity to use the artificial airways alongside my expertise with the heart-lung machine.

In 1992, I was invited to the Cape Town conference to celebrate the twenty-fifth anniversary of Christiaan Barnard's first heart transplant. At that meeting, the distinguished children's heart surgeon Susan Vosloo asked me to see a sick two-year-old who had been a patient at the Red Cross War Memorial Children's Hospital for several weeks. Little Oslin lived in the sprawling Cape Town ghetto situated between the airport and the city, acre upon acre of tin shacks, wooden sheds, and tents with brackish water and little sanitation. Nevertheless, he was a cheerful little chap. His toys were oil drums, tin cans, and pieces of wood. He knew no other life.

One day the family's faulty gas cylinder exploded in the shack, setting fire to the walls and roof. The blast killed Oslin's father. Oslin sustained severe burns to his face and chest. Worse still, he inhaled hot gas from the blast. Much like Mario. The Accident Department at Red Cross saved his life. They intubated and ventilated him before he asphyxiated, then treated the burns with intravenous fluids and antibiotics. The boy could survive the external burns. More worrying were the burned-out trachea and main bronchi. On top of that, his face was badly disfigured and he was almost blind. He couldn't swallow food, only saliva. So he was fed with liquids through a tube directly into the stomach.

It happened that Dr. Susan Vosloo had read the journal article about Mario and the tube I had designed. Although Oslin was much smaller, she wondered whether we could do anything to help him. When I first met the boy, he was pushing himself around the ward on a kiddie bicycle. He had his back to me. He was wearing a bright-red shirt and had tight curly black hair. Susan called to him and he turned around. The sight took my breath away. There was no hair on the front of his scalp. No eyelids, just white sclera and severely burned nose and lips. His neck was webbed from contracting scars, with a tracheostomy tube in the middle. And the noise was heart-rending. He was rattling with thick mucus secretions. You could hear a long, noisy drawing-in of breath followed by a high-pitched wheeze as he forcibly exhaled. It was worse than a horror movie and tragic beyond belief. My immediate thought was: *Poor kid, he should have died with his dad. It would have been much kinder.*

Strangely enough, he seemed happy. He had never had a bicycle before the explosion. I kneeled on the floor to talk with him. He looked straight at me, but I couldn't tell whether he could see my face. His corneas were opaque. So I took his little hand. There would be no objectivity in this discussion. I needed to help him. Even if I wasn't sure how it could be done. We could work that out.

By then I was the chief of cardiac surgery at Oxford's John Radcliffe Hospital. I had to get back there to operate. In any case, there was no "Westaby Tube" in Cape Town. And even if there were, it wouldn't have fit—the adult size was too big. Could I persuade the company to make a smaller tube? Probably not within the time limits that we faced. If he developed pneumonia in the next couple of weeks, he would surely die.

I was scheduled to fly back to Heathrow the following day. Instead of going for lunch on the harbor, I asked Susan whether she would take me to see Oslin's township. Cape Town was my favorite city in the world, but this was a side of it I had never seen before. It was the sort of place that warranted an armed escort. Thousands of acres of misery and depravity. I decided to return in a couple of weeks, when I had the tube and a surgical strategy. That's what flying time was for. Soon I had it clear in my mind. Before the wheels touched down in Heathrow, I had drawn the operation in detail.

Three weeks later, I was back in the Children's Hospital. They had already held a fund-raising drive to help Oslin. They expected to pay my expenses. But none of that mattered. I was driven to help the boy. No kid on earth deserved to live in such a state. In spite of our brief acquaintance, I cared deeply about Oslin. So did the doctors and nurses at Red Cross. Perhaps the whole of Cape Town. As the airport taxi reached the city, I saw the newspaper billboards. They said: "UK Doc Flies In to Save Township Boy." On lamppost after lamppost. No pressure then.

It was then that I met Oslin's mother for the first time. She had been at work when the gas cylinder exploded. She was clearly distressed and said virtually nothing. She signed the consent form for an operation that even I didn't understand.

We operated the following morning. I had to trim the adult tube by shortening both bronchial limbs, the tracheostomy T-piece and the top part that would sit below his vocal cords. Still, this shortened adult tube would not fit inside the two-year-old's scarred windpipe. My objective was to rebuild his major airways around the tube. If it worked, he would have even wider airways than before the accident. It was clear he wouldn't be able to breathe or be ventilated during the reconstructive surgery. We would do it with the support of the heart-lung machine. This meant we would have to open his sternum as we would in a heart operation. The tricky part was to gain access to the whole length of the trachea and main bronchial tubes from an incision in the front of his chest. These structures were situated directly behind the heart and large blood vessels.

I had worked the logistics out on a cadaver in the medical school dissecting room in Oxford. When a sling was placed around the aorta and the adjacent superior vena cava, they could be pulled apart to expose the back of the pericardial sac, like opening a pair of curtains and looking out onto a tree. Then a vertical incision between the two served to expose the lower trachea and both main bronchi. My plan was to fillet these damaged tubes, then lay in the modified T-Y stent. We would then repair the front of the opened airways and cover the tube with a patch of Oslin's own pericardium, like sewing an elbow patch onto a worn jacket sleeve. Simple. It should all heal up around the tube. In time, maybe we could remove the prosthesis. After the tissues had healed and molded around the silicone. Anyway, that was my plan. Maybe "fantasy" would have been a more accurate term, but no one else had a better solution.

The skin incision started in Oslin's neck, just below his voice box. It extended all the way down to the cartilage at the lower end of the breastbone. There was no fat. The electrocautery cut straight through to the bone. Then we sawed through that. I cut out the fleshy, redundant thymus gland and dissected down onto the upper part of the inflamed trachea. He was ventilated through his tracheostomy tube. We needed to go on bypass before removing this and exposing the rest of the airways. The metal retractor stretched open his scarred little chest, exposing more of the fibrous pericardium. The front of this was removed for the tracheal patch. His little heart was beating happily away. Rarely do I see a normal child's heart. Most are deformed and struggling.

When I was ready to open the windpipe, we started the bypass machine. This rendered the lungs redundant so we could remove the contaminated tracheostomy tube from the clean surgical field. Through the hole, the devastation was clear to see. Poor Oslin had been breathing through a sewer. I cut down the length of it with the electrocautery and continued the incision into each main bronchus until I could see normal respiratory lining at the limits of our access. Copious thick secretions poured out of the obstructed airways. Then we scraped tissue off the walls, with predicable bleeding. As the cautery eventually stopped the hemorrhage, we laid in the shiny white T-Y tube and covered over it with the patch of

Oslin's own pericardium. I adjusted the length of the rubber cylinder for the last time. Striving for perfection. And obsessively sewed the patch into place to seal the implant. It needed to be airtight, otherwise the ventilator would push air into the tissues of the neck and chest. Then he would blow up like the Michelin man. With the shiny new breathing tubes attached to the ventilator, we blew air into his little lungs. There was no leak. Both inflated and then deflated normally. A sense of excitement permeated the room. The high-risk strategy was working.

Oslin's heart bounced off the bypass machine. His lungs moved freely, needing much lower pressure from the ventilator. Our anesthetist murmured "unbelievable. I would never have believed it possible." I covered the repair by closing the back wall of his pericardium, then asked that the resident put in the drains and close.

Oslin's mother was sitting in the ICU waiting room. We could see her through the window. Still, expressionless, and rigid with fear. A portrait of mental anguish in a tormented life. I anticipated a blunt response to our news. She was too emotionally drained to register relief. She simply held out her hand and squeezed mine. She murmured, "God bless you." A tear zigzagged down her pock-marked cheek. I wished her a better life in the future.

The ICU was pleased to have Oslin back. Most of the patients there were township kids having heart surgery. Some of the nurses lived in that same environment. They had cared for Oslin and his depressed mom for weeks, watching them both deteriorate. So "UK Doc" had succeeded in saving township boy. I was proud of that. Now it was time to ride off into the sunset.

Oslin recovered and could breathe freely through the white rubber tube in his neck. He couldn't speak but went on to have his corneal transplants. Being able to breathe and see at the same time was as much as he could have hoped for. The little family was relocated to better social housing on the outskirts of the city, their environment crude but clean and safer. He was still vulnerable, however—a chest infection could still kill him.

For the first few months afterward, I contacted Cape Town frequently. Oslin was doing fine. Mom was faring better on anti-depressants. Then I stopped calling.

Eighteen months later, a letter arrived from the Red Cross Hospital. Oslin had been found dead at home. No one knew why. Sometimes, life is shit.

five   The Girl with No Name

Dream that my little baby came to life again; that it had only been cold, and that we rubbed it before the fire, and it lived. Awake and find no baby.

—Mary Shelley

THE GIRL WAS HAUNTINGLY BEAUTIFUL, WITH EYES THAT burned like lasers. As if the blistering desert heat was not enough. One hundred and twenty-two degrees Fahrenheit during the day. When she fixed those eyes on mine, she delivered a message. Pupil to pupil. Retina to retina, then in to my cerebral cortex. As she stood there holding her bundle of rags, I understood perfectly what she was saying: "Please save my child." But she never spoke. Not to any of us. Ever. We never knew her name.

The Kingdom of Saudi Arabia, 1987. Thirty years ago. I was young and fearless. Seemingly invincible and massively overconfident. I had just been appointed in Oxford. So why was I in the desert? Heart operations cost money. We had worked hard to build a new cardiac center and clear a backlog of sick hearts. Yet the annual budget was gone in five months. So the management closed us down. Forget the patients. The cardiologists were told to send them to London.

The day before I was locked out of the operating theater, I took a call from a prestigious Saudi cardiac center that served the entire Arab world. The center's lead surgeon needed three months' sick leave. They were looking for a temp who could tackle both congenital and adult heart surgery. An increasingly rare species even then. Yesterday I wasn't interested. Today I was. Three days later I was on a plane.

It was Jumadath-Thaniyya, the "Second Month of Dryness" in the Middle East. I had never felt anything like it. Blistering, unremitting heat, with the hot Shamal wind blowing sand into the city. But it was home to a great cardiac center. My medical colleagues were an eclectic mix of Saudi men who had trained overseas, Americans rotating from the major centers for experience, and a band of mercenaries from Europe and Australasia. Nursing was different. Saudi women did not nurse. The profession was regarded with suspicion and disrespect, and it was culturally off-limits because it required mixing with the opposite sex. So all nurses were foreign. Most had contracts for one or two years. Their accommodation was free, they paid no tax and stayed just long enough to save for that mortgage back home. In turn they were not allowed to drive, had to travel in the rear of buses, and had to be completely covered in public.

I was intrigued by my new environment. The repeated calls for prayer from the minarets. The tantalizing aromas of sandalwood, incense, and amber around the hospital. Arabian coffee roasting on the frying pan or boiling with cardamom. It was a very different life, and yet I was keenly aware that I could not step out of line. Their culture, their rules, harsh penalties for all.

Professionally, this presented a unique opportunity. I could operate on every conceivable congenital anomaly. There were innumerable young patients with rheumatic heart disease sent from remote towns and villages, mostly without access to anticoagulant therapy or drugs that we take for granted in the West. Their rural health care was from the Middle Ages. We had to innovate and improvise to repair their heart valves rather than replace them with prosthetic materials. I remember thinking that every cardiac surgeon should train here.

One morning, a bright young pediatric cardiologist from the Mayo Clinic, the world-famous medical center in Minnesota, came to find me in the operating theater. "Can I show you something interesting?" he asked. "Bet you haven't seen anything like this before." He continued, "Sadly, I doubt you can do anything about it." I was immediately determined to prove him wrong before I had even seen the case. Presented with unique specimens, surgeons can resemble kids with a new toy. The unusual is always a challenge.

He thrust the X-ray onto a light box. On a plain chest X-ray, the heart is simply a gray shadow. Yet to the educated eye it can tell a story. The message was clear. This was a small child with an enlarged heart pointing toward the wrong side of the chest, a rare anomaly called dextrocardia. Normal hearts lie to the left. And there was fluid on the lungs. Dextrocardia alone does not cause heart failure. There had to be another problem.

The enthusiastic Mayo cardiologist was testing me. He had already catheterized the eighteen-month-old boy and knew the answer. I offered an insightful guess to show off. "In this part of the world it could be Lutembacher syndrome." This is a dextrocardia heart with a large hole between the right and left atrium, together with rheumatic fever that narrows the mitral valve. The rare combination floods the lungs with blood, leaving the rest of the body short. The Mayo man was impressed. But no cigar! Now he wanted to take me to see the angiogram, a moving X-ray picture with dye shot into the circulation to clarify the anatomy. By now I was growing annoyed with the quizzing, but I went along. There was a huge sinister mass within the cavity of the left ventricle below the aortic valve. Almost cutting off the flow of blood around the body. I could see this was a tumor. Whether benign or malignant, the infant could not survive for much longer. Could I remove it?

I had never seen surgery on a dextrocardia heart before. Most never would. But I knew about heart tumors in children. I had published a paper on the subject. The pediatric cardiologist had read it and that made me the expert on the subject in Saudi Arabia.

The most common tumor in babies is a benign mass of abnormal heart muscle and fibrous tissue called a rhabdomyoma. Often these are associated with a brain abnormality that causes epileptic fits. No one knew whether the boy had suffered fits, but he was certainly dying from an obstructed heart. I asked the child's age and whether his parents understood the desperate nature of the condition. Then the tragic story began to unfold.

It happened that the boy and his young mother were close to death when the Red Cross found them on the border between Oman and South Yemen. In the searing heat, both were emaciated, dehydrated, and in a state of collapse. Apparently, this mother had carried her son through the desert and mountains of Yemen, frantic to seek medical help. They were airlifted to the Military Hospital in Muscat in Oman, where they found that she was still trying to breastfeed. She had nothing else to feed her son, but her milk had dried up. When rehydrated with fluids into a vein the boy became breathless and was diagnosed with heart failure. In turn, the mother had severe abdominal pain and a high temperature from pelvic infection. Yemen was lawless. She had been raped, abused, and mutilated. Not only that, she was African, not Arabic. The Red Cross suspected that she had been kidnapped from Somalia and taken across the Gulf of Aden to be sold as a slave. But they couldn't be sure. She never spoke. Not a word. And she barely showed emotion, even in response to pain.

When the Omanis saw the boy's chest X-ray and diagnosed dextrocardia and heart failure, they transferred him to our hospital.

Now, the Mayo man wondered whether I could conjure up a miracle. I knew that the Mayo had a great children's heart surgeon, so I tentatively asked my colleague what Dr. Danielson would do. "Operate, I guess," the cardiologist said in response. "Unless we do, it's all downhill from here." That's what I expected him to say.

What else did I need to know about the boy? Not only was his heart in the wrong side of the chest, but the abdominal organs were switched over, too. What we call *situs inversus*. The liver was in the left upper quadrant of the belly with the stomach and the spleen on the right. The bigger problem was that there was a large hole between the left atrium and right atrium. So blood returning from both the body and the veins of the lungs mixed freely. This meant that the level of oxygen in the arteries to his body was lower than it should be. Had his skin not been black, he might have been recognized as a "blue baby," with blood in the veins streaming across into the arteries. Complicated stuff even for doctors.

Money was no object here. We had state-of-the-art echocardiography, which in those days was new and exciting, based on ultrasound waves used to detect submarines under water. An accomplished operator could provide sharp pictures of the inside of the heart and measure pressure gradients across areas of obstruction. It gave a clear image of the tumor in the small left ventricle. Smooth and round, like a bantam's egg. I felt confident that it was benign; it would not grow back, if only I could relieve him of it.

My plan was to clear the obstruction and close the hole in the heart, an ambitious attempt to restore normal physiology. Straightforward in principle yet taxing in a back-to-front heart in the wrong side of the chest. I didn't want any surprises, so I did what I always do in difficult circumstances and set about to draw the anatomy in detail.

Was the surgery possible? I didn't know, but we had to try. Even if we failed to remove the tumor completely, it would still help him. Although should it prove to be a rare malignancy, his outlook was bleak.

It was time to meet the boy and his mother. Mayo man took me to the pediatric high-dependency unit, where he was still being fed via a tube through his nose, which he disliked intensely. The mother was sitting cross-legged on a mat on the floor beside the child's bed. She never left his side. At night, she slept there.

As we approached, she rose up. Not what I expected. She was stunningly beautiful, with a striking resemblance to David Bowie's Somali model wife, Iman. Her jet-black hair was straight and long, her skinny arms folded across her chest. The Red Cross had established that she was Somali. A Christian, so her head was not covered.

Her long, delicate fingers were clutching the bundle in which she held her son. Precious rags that had shielded him from the hot sun, then kept him warm in the cold desert nights. An umbilical cord of drip tubing emerged from these swaddling clothes, stretching to the drip pole and a bottle of feed. Milky white solution replete with glucose, amino acids, vitamins, and minerals. To put meat back on his little bones.

Her eyes turned toward the stranger, the English heart surgeon whom she had heard about. Her head gently tilted backward in an attempt to remain detached. A bead of sweat appeared in the root of her neck and slithered down over the sternal notch. She was growing anxious.

I tried to engage with her in Arabic. "*Sabah al Khair*"—Good morning. "*Aysh ismuk*"—What is your name? She said nothing and looked at the floor. Showing off unmercifully, I said "*Terref arabi*"—Do you know Arabic? Then "*Inta min weyn*"—Where are you from? Still no response. Finally in desperation I uttered "*Titakellem ingleezi*"—Do you speak English? "*Ana min ingliterra*"—I am from England. Then she looked up, wide eyed, and I knew that she understood. Her lips parted but still no words. She was mute. Mayo man was speechless, too, stunned by my language skills, which unbeknownst to him had been just about exhausted. She appeared to appreciate my efforts.

Her shoulders dropped. She relaxed. I wanted to show her kindness, to take her hand, but I couldn't in this environment.

I indicated that I would like to examine the boy. That was fine as long as she could continue to hold him. I was shocked as she pulled back his linen covering. The little fellow was emaciated, all his ribs protruding. There was virtually no fat on him, and I could see his bizarre heart pounding against his chest wall. He was breathing rapidly to overcome the stiffness in his lungs. His protuberant belly was full of fluid, with the enlarged liver clearly visible on the opposite side to normal. From the different skin tone, I assumed that the father was Arabic. A curious rash covered his dark olive skin, and his little brown eyes stared into the distance. As if I wasn't there. Then I knew that she was losing him.

The mother pulled the linens back over his face, protectively. He was all she had in the world. The boy and a few rags and rings. I couldn't help the surge of pity I felt for both of them. Surgery was my business, but I was sucked into this whirlpool of despair. My objectivity gone. Too much of my own testosterone.

In those days I had a red stethoscope. I placed it on the infant's chest, trying to look professional. There was a harsh murmur as blood squeezed past the tumor and out through the aortic valve. Then the crackling sounds of wet lungs. Even the gurgling and bubbling of empty guts. The cacophony of the human body.

Next I said *"Mumken asaduq"*—roughly translated, "Will you let me help you?" For a second I thought she responded. Her lips moved. Those eyes fixed on mine. I thought she murmured, *"Naam"*—yes. I tried to explain that I needed to operate on the boy's heart, to make him well. So they both could have a better life. When tears appeared in her eyes, I knew that she understood.

We managed to get her to sign the consent form, all in silence, our eyes still locked together. I was searching for approval, I guess. By now her skin was glistening with perspiration. She was pouring out adrenaline. Trembling with anxiety.

It was time for us to leave her alone. I indicated that I would do the operation on Sunday when I had the best pediatric anesthetist. Then I said good-bye in both English and Arabic.

This was Thursday afternoon. The day before the Saudi weekend. My colleagues were planning to take me out for a night in the desert. Camping on the dunes beneath the night sky. It was a way of escaping the oppression of the city. The convoy left late in the afternoon, just as the searing heat started to abate. When we ran out of road, the jeeps plowed through the sand. Miles and miles of it. They had a rule—never travel in only one vehicle. If it broke down that could be the end, even within twenty miles of the hospital.

The desert night was clear and cold. We sat around the campfire drinking homemade hooch and watching shooting stars. A Bedouin camel train passed by silently two hundred yards away, Kalashnikovs and swords glinting in the moonlight. Intimidating, but they didn't even acknowledge us.

I felt uneasy. I wondered how the girl had coped, walking at night, hoping to find shelter during the day. Carrying water and child together. Fueled by hope but little else. However difficult it proved to be, I was driven to save the child and watch them both grow stronger.

I knew that the operation would be far from straightforward. I was still unsure how to get at this tumor. In a small heart, the obstruction would only be accessible by widely opening the apex of the left ventricle, and that would impair its pumping ability. I kept working through the steps of the operation in my mind. Repeatedly coming back to the question "What if?" With conventional surgery the technical challenges posed by the dextrocardia heart were virtually insurmountable. Would the child be better off operated on by a more experienced surgeon in America? I couldn't see why, because the combination of pathologies was probably unique. No one else would have greater experience, even if they had a better team. I had a good enough team. And great equipment. So I was the man for the job. Wasn't I? It was then that I had my eureka moment—while staring at the Milky Way. I knew how to get at the tumor. Obvious, but perhaps outrageous. I had a plan.

On Saturday evening, I succeeded in bringing the anesthetic and surgical teams together to discuss the case. I showed them the novel pictures of the unusual anatomy. Then I told them the girl's heartrending story. So much of what happens in an operating theater remains impersonal. Which is perhaps best when operating on those who may not survive. Everyone agreed that the child was doomed if we made no effort. Then they expressed justifiable concerns that the tumor was inoperable in dextrocardia. I said that we would only know that through trying, but I kept the operating plan to myself.

I spent a hot, restless night in the apartment, my mind racing, disturbed by irrational thoughts. Would I have risked this back in England? Was I doing it for the patient or the mother? Or for myself so I could publish a paper about it? If I succeeded, who would care for this slave girl and her illegitimate child? The boy was an inconvenience. In Yemen, he would be left out under a bush for the wolves to eat. It was the mother they wanted. Perhaps I did, too.

The early morning call to prayer put an end to my discomfort. It was already 83°F as I walked from the apartment to the hospital. Mother and son came down to the operating theater complex and anesthetic room at 7:00 a.m. She had stayed awake with the child in her arms. All night long the nurses had been worried that she might run away. She didn't, but they were still concerned about whether she would hand the boy over. Despite premedication, he was screaming when they tried to put him to sleep. Thrashing around. Dreadful for the mother. Difficult for the anesthetic staff but pretty much routine in pediatric surgery. Gas through the face mask eventually subdued him enough to insert a cannula into a vein and stun him into unconsciousness. She wanted to follow him into the operating theater. The ward nurses eventually dragged her away. Finally, raw emotion broke through the mask. Whatever she had suffered physically, this was worse. Still, there were no words.

I sat dispassionate in the coffee room until the mayhem abated. Thick Turkish coffee and dates for breakfast. The caffeine load was good for my attention deficit disorder but racked up my sense of responsibility. What if the child dies? Then she has nothing.

One of the Australian scrub nurses came through to ask that I check the equipment—the extra things I had requested for my radical option conceived in the desert. I had yet to share it with my team.

Uncovered on the shiny black vinyl of an operating table, this starved little body was a pathetic sight. There was none of the puppy fat that every infant deserves. Instead, his skinny legs were swollen with fluid. The heart failure paradox. Muscle replaced by water but weight stays the same. Prominent ribs rising and falling with the ventilator. No longer struggling for breath on his own. Now everyone understood why the mother was so fiercely protective. We could see the heart beating away in the wrong side of the chest and the outline of his swollen liver in the contrary side of the bulging abdomen. Everything reversed. A source of fascination for the onlookers; a daunting challenge for me. I had seen one operation on dextrocardia in the United States and another at Great Ormond Street Hospital. This would be the first I had attempted myself.

There were still streaks of dried salt down his cheeks from the traumatic separation. What was it I used to say? When asked if I was ever anxious about undertaking an operation. "No. It's not me on the table!" I don't do anxiety. But now I was in tiger country with an untested procedure in an unfamiliar environment. I could feel sweat trickling down my back. It felt a long way from Oxford.

Everyone was relieved when that fragile little body was covered in blue drapes, leaving only a rectangular window of dark skin exposed over the breastbone. He was not a child anymore, just a surgical challenge. Until we heard the tormented mother banging on the operating theater doors. She had given her minders the slip and rushed back. After a struggle, they allowed her to sit in the corridor outside. Her day was traumatic enough without being dragged away for a second time.

The scalpel blade slid along the length of the sternum. Left to right until a trickle of bright-red blood skidded over the plastic drape. The electrocautery soon put a stop to that as it sizzled down onto white bone. The whiff of white smoke told me that the diathermy had too much power. I reminded the orderly that we were operating on a child, not electing a pope, so would he please turn down the voltage.

Heart failure fluid was pushing up the diaphragm. I made a small hole in the abdominal cavity. Straw-colored fluid poured out like piss into the wound. The noisy sucker removed almost a pint into the drainage bottle, and the belly flattened out. A quick way to lose weight. The saw zipped up the sternum, spraying beads of bone marrow onto the plastic. It breached the right chest cavity, releasing a knuckle of stiff, pink, waterlogged lung. Still more fluid spilled out, and the sucker bottle had to be changed. It left no one in any doubt that this kid was seriously unwell.

Impatient to view the congenitally distorted heart, I dissected away the thymus gland and sliced open the pericardium, the fibrous sac that encases the heart. Everyone wanted to get a good look at the dextrocardia heart before I started. So I took a step back and relaxed for a minute.

The plan was to open up the narrowed channel below the aortic valve by coring out as much solid tumor as possible, then close the hole in the atrial septum. I gave the order to go onto the heart-lung machine and proceeded to stop the empty heart with cardioplegia fluid. It lay cold, still, and flaccid in the bottom of the pericardial sac. I gently palpated the muscle and could feel the rubbery tumor through the heart wall. By now I was sure that I couldn't reach it all with a conventional approach. There was little point in cutting into the ventricle that his circulation depended upon purely on an exploratory basis. There was only one choice left. Plan B. The option I'd hit upon that night. In those days, it had probably never been done before. The perfusionist began to cool the whole body down from 98°F to 82°F. The boy was likely to be on the bypass machine for at least two hours.

At that point, I had to share my outlandish plan with the rest of the team. I would cut out the boy's heart from the chest and operate on it on the bench. Lying on a kidney dish full of ice to keep it cool. Then I could twist and turn the thing as much as I needed to do a good job. Brilliant. At least I thought so, and from the team's stunned reaction, I felt that they agreed! But I had to work fast.

The process was equivalent to removing a donor heart for transplant, then sewing it back into the same patient. Back in my research days, I had transplanted tiny rat hearts. This child's heart should not be a problem, even with its unusual anatomy. So I began. I transected the aorta just beyond the origin of the coronary arteries. Then the main pulmonary artery. By pulling these vessels toward me, the roof of the left atrium was exposed at the back of this heart. I cut through the atria, leaving all the large veins from the body and lungs in place, lifting the ventricles out and leaving most of the atria in situ. As one would for a donor heart, I placed the cold, floppy muscle onto the ice.

Now I could see the tumor within the outflow part of the left ventricle. I started to dissect it out; to cut a channel through it so that it would no longer obstruct the heart. The rubbery texture was consistent with it being benign, making me optimistic that we had done the right thing. Both my assistants were shocked and mesmerized by the empty chest. They were not assisting well. And the longer this heart was without a blood supply, the more likely it would fail when I re-implanted it. Thankfully, the Australian scrub nurse was much sharper than these trainees, so I asked her to help. She knew instinctively what was required and injected the necessary pace into the procedure.

I was torn between just doing enough or making a radical job of it. I wanted to tell his mother that I had succeeded in removing it all. So I pursued the tumor into the ventricular septum, close to the heart's electrical wiring system. I knew where this was situated in a normal heart. Its location was less certain in this case. After thirty minutes I infused another dose of cardioplegia solution directly into both coronary arteries, to keep the heart cold and flaccid. In another fifteen minutes the job was done. I took it back to his body, aligned the ventricles with the atrial cuffs, and started to sew it in. Really impressed with myself. The journal publication half written in my head. The re-implantation process also closed the hole in the heart so the child was cured. Or so I hoped.

This part of the operation had to be fail-safe. In the beating heart, these stitch lines would be inaccessible. With both atria joined up, it was time to reattach the aorta and let blood back into the coronary arteries. The heart would start beating again, and we could rewarm the whole child. All that was left was to reattach the main pulmonary artery. By then the surgical assistants had also warmed up a bit. Back to familiar territory with the heart where it belonged.

Usually a child's heart starts to beat spontaneously and fast when its blood flow is restored. This one was too slow. What's more, I could see that the atria and the ventricles were contracting at different rates. This told me that the conduction system between the two was not working. The anesthetist had already noticed this on the electrocardiogram but said nothing. After cooling, the conduction system often goes to sleep for a while and then recovers spontaneously. Coordinated heart rhythm is much more efficient. Ten minutes later and nothing had changed. I must have cut through the electrical bundle while dissecting out the tumor. Dammit. He would need a pacemaker. This made me anxious about another issue. A transplanted heart also loses its connection with nerves from the brain. Nerves that automatically speed up or slow down the heart during exercise or changes in blood volume. This denervation, together with disruption of the electrical conduction system, could be a real problem.

My euphoria and optimism abated. The young mother drifted back into my thoughts. Not a good time to lose focus. There was still air within the heart chambers and it had to be let out. I inserted a hollow needle into the aorta and pulmonary artery. Air fizzed out from both. When air entered the uppermost right coronary artery, the right ventricle distended and stopped pumping. We needed another fifteen minutes on the bypass machine for the effects to wear off. During that time, I put temporary pacing electrodes on the right atrium and ventricle. We would control his heart rate with these wires until the cardiologists could implant a permanent pacemaker. Gradually the heart function improved. Obstruction gone, lungs relieved of congestion. Life relieved of heart failure and breathlessness. Or so I hoped.

The boy's pulse rate was only forty beats per minute, less than half what it should be. We increased that to ninety beats per minute with the external pacemaker. With this improvement, blood started to well up from behind the heart. Persistent bleeding, which I assumed was leaking through my stitching. I told the perfusionist to turn the bypass machine off and empty the heart while I lifted it up to inspect the join. Nothing. It looked great. No leak. When we restarted the machine, thirty seconds later there was more blood. I inspected the joins of the aorta and pulmonary artery. No leak. Eventually my first assistant spotted oozing from the aorta. The needle used to evacuate air had penetrated the back wall. A small hole, which would be inconsequential when blood clotting was restored. So we separated from the heart-lung machine and closed the chest.

I didn't have long to reflect on the success. There was another message. This time from the adult cardiologists. They had admitted a young male following a high-speed road-traffic accident. Without a seat belt, his chest had impacted against the steering wheel with great force. He was in shock and his blood pressure could not be restored by fluid resuscitation. Chest X-rays at the referring hospital had shown a fractured sternum and an enlarged heart shadow. The veins in his neck were distended, suggesting blood under pressure in the pericardial sac. Not only that. The echocardiogram showed that the tricuspid valve, between right atrium and ventricle, was leaking badly. Hence the persistently low blood pressure and severe shock. The man needed urgent surgery. Could I please come and see him before it was too late?

I was distinctly uneasy about leaving the child, but there was no choice. Leaving the operating theater complex, I found the mother sitting cross-legged in the corridor. She had been waiting there for five hours. Alone and desolate. I sensed that she was about to implode mentally. She had bottled up her emotions for too long. Unable to communicate. And we had taken away her bundle of rags. She saw me, sprang to her feet and panicked. Was the operation a success? I didn't need to speak. The eyes met again. Pupil to pupil. Retina to retina. My smile was enough. With it the message that her son was still alive.

Screw protocol and the audience of cardiologists. I needed to show her some affection. I held out a sticky hand, wondering whether she would take it or remain aloof. This act of kindness unlocked the tension. She took it and began to shake uncontrollably. I pulled her in and held her tight. As if to say, You are safe now. We won't let anyone harm you anymore. When I let go, she held on and started to weep uncontrollably. Waves of emotion discharged on the hospital corridor, leaving my Saudi colleagues standing in an embarrassed silence. It took a while to calm her. They were becoming increasingly anxious about their trauma patient.

I told her that her son would shortly leave the operating theater and that they would wheel him out in an intensive-care bed, attached to drips and drains that would frighten her. She could walk with them but not interfere. Again I sensed that she understood

English. The cardiologists repeated my words in Arabic. Then we left to review the injured man's echocardiograms.

By now the trauma patient was dying. He had a rare high-speed deceleration injury. A torn tricuspid valve. Something we never see with seat belts. The right ventricle was pulverized when the sternum fractured and was driven back against the spine. The rapid increase in pressure had caused the valve to burst. Now when the heart contracted as much blood went backward as forward. Little was passing through the lungs. And the heart couldn't fill adequately because of blood in the pericardium. "Cardiac tamponade," we call it.

Once I had seen the pictures I didn't waste time visiting the patient. I needed to open him up, relieve the tamponade, and if possible repair the tricuspid valve. We needed to get onto the heart-lung machine quickly to restore blood flow to the brain and correct his dire metabolic state. Then someone behind me whispered, "Don't rush. He's a madman. He killed the other driver." I said nothing. That wasn't my business. Striding purposefully back to the operating theater, I encountered the little entourage in transit to the pediatric ICU. The fast regular beeping of the heart-rate monitor was reassuring. Without diverting her gaze, the mother held out her hand as we crossed over. I did the same. Contact.

I should have been with the child in the ICU. At least for the first couple of hours. Until I was confident that he was stable. But now I couldn't be. Soon the man was on the operating table being resuscitated. He had disfiguring facial injuries and extensive bruising over the chest wall. The edges of the fractured sternum overlapped. Nothing we couldn't fix with pins and wires. Within minutes I had the chest and pericardium open and was scooping clumps of blood clot into a kidney dish. This improved the blood pressure, but his right ventricle looked like tenderized steak. The right atrium was distended to the bursting point. So I put the pipes directly into the major veins. As we started cardiopulmonary bypass (CPB), the struggling heart emptied out and flapped around at the bottom of the pericardial sac. Like a wet fish. Just in time, he was safe. With an incision directly into the right atrium, the ruptured valve was there in front of me. Torn like a curtain. Stitched like cloth and easily repaired. I tested it by filling the right ventricle through a bulb syringe. No leak. So I closed the atrium and removed the snares to fill it again. The job was done. The tenderized meat functioned better than anticipated and eased itself off the bypass machine. By then, I had had enough. I left my assistants to repair the fractured sternum and close the chest. No doubt he would survive to go to prison.

The sun was setting on a hot and difficult day. For a while I felt content. Satisfied after two "out-on-the-edge" operations. Difficult cases that most heart surgeons would never encounter in their whole career. I needed a beer. Many beers, but no chance of that. I wondered, was the girl happier now? She had achieved what she set out for—treatment for her dying child.

Having heard nothing from the ICU, I assumed that the child was doing fine. Wrong. They were already in trouble. For some reason, the doctors had tampered with the temporary pacing box. The electric stimulus from the generator had coincided with a natural beat and fibrillated the heart, that incoordinate squirming rhythm that heralds imminent death. They had used external cardiac massage until a defibrillator was brought to the bedside. The vigorous chest compressions had displaced the pacing wire from the atrium. Although the heart defibrillated at the first shock, the sequential pacing of atrium, then ventricle, no longer worked. Only the ventricles could be paced. As a result there was a precipitous drop in cardiac output. The kidneys had stopped working. The child was deteriorating, but no one had told me. Because I was in the middle of another big case.

Throughout this debacle, the poor mother had stayed by the bed. She watched them pounding on her little boy's chest. Then applying the electrical shock that caused his little body to spring from the bed and convulse. At least he only needed one shot at defibrillation. The resulting beep, beep, beep, was of little comfort to her. Like the child, she was spiraling down.

I found her clasping his tiny hand, tears running down her cheeks. She had been happy as she escorted him from the operating theater. Now she was desolate. So was I. It was clear that these intensive-care doctors didn't understand cardiac transplant physiology. Why should they? They had never been involved with heart transplants. They failed to grasp that taking the heart out cut off its normal nerve supply. They were pacing the heart at 100 beats per minute with insufficient blood volume. At the same time they were flogging the heart with high doses of adrenaline to raise the blood pressure. This constricted the arteries to his muscles and organs, substituting blood pressure for flow, producing metabolic mayhem.

The nurse looking after the boy on the ICU ward was anxious and relieved to see me. A capable New Zealander, she clearly did not rate the critical-care resident. She immediately said, "He's not passing urine and they're not doing anything about it." The next comment was more direct. "If you're not careful, they're going to fuck up your good work!" I put my hand on the child's leg—the best way to judge cardiac output. The feet should be warm, with bounding pulses. They were cold.

He needed dilated arteries, less resistance to flow, and less demand for oxygen. So I changed everything. Now the nurse was happier, but the resident was put out. He phoned the on-call attending physician. That was fine. I told the attending physician to get himself in from home and discuss it.

We now walked the delicate path between recovery and death. Much depended upon expert management. Minute by minute. Beat by beat. Balancing the cocktail of powerful drugs. Maximizing this compromised little heart's pumping capacity. The lungs were inflamed and stiff after the long period on the heart-lung machine. So the oxygen levels in his blood were falling. Already the kidney failure warranted dialysis through a catheter inserted into the abdominal cavity. Using concentrated fluids to draw the poisons out through the child's own membranes. I needed the help of someone I could trust. Mayo man. I would stay in one of the on-call rooms, which were a couple of minutes away from where the residents slept.

The mother didn't want me to leave. Tears flowed over those high cheekbones. Her profound separation anxiety was trying to pull me back. But by then I was physically exhausted. And fearful of how it would be if the child died. She had no one else in the world. Although I wanted to be kind, it was time to take a step backward. Call it professionalism or self-protection. Perhaps both. I reassured her that Mayo man was on his way. Then I left.

By now it was well after midnight. The on-call rooms overlooked the rooftops. The clubroom opened onto a veranda under the night sky. Not as spectacular as the sand dunes at night, but good enough. There was sustenance: juice, coffee, olives, and dates. And Arab pastries. Best of all, a telescope for stargazing. I looked out at nothing in particular, wishing I could see England and home. Most of all my little family.

Now I tried to switch off. Mayo man knew I had more babies to operate on in the morning. They would only call me if absolutely necessary. I was desperate to find an improving child. With hot little legs and liquid gold in the urinary catheter. And I wanted to see her happy. Cradling her boy in rags again.

I passed out in a heap. In my mind those deeply penetrating eyes still fixed on me. Pleading with me to make things right.

Chanting from the minarets roused me at dawn. Around 5:30 a.m. The fact that there was no night call from the ICU was reason for guarded optimism. Today's operations were easy enough. Holes in the heart to be closed with a cloth patch. Careful stitching, and then cured for life. Happy parents.

I was thinking about the girl. How was she feeling now? I soon found out that she felt nothing. I took tea out onto the roof as the blistering sun hauled itself into the sky. The temperature was bearable, the air still cool and fresh.

At 6:00 a.m., Mayo man called. After a pause he said, "Sorry to wake you with bad news. The boy died just after 3:00 a.m. Quite suddenly. We couldn't get him back." Then silence in anticipation of my questions. I had had calls like this my whole career, but this one made me especially miserable. He recounted what had happened. At first the boy started fitting. Perhaps in response to the metabolic mess and high temperature. Violent fits that were difficult to control with barbiturate drugs. The acid and potassium in his blood were still high because dialysis had not been started yet. When he had a cardiac arrest, they couldn't get him back. Mayo man was hesitant to wake me when I had more babies to operate on today. You could tell he was sorry.

My thoughts immediately turned to the mother. Did they want me to come across and try to communicate with her? Mayo man didn't think that would do any good. Again she had been by the bed during the resuscitation efforts and was distressed. Hysterical beyond reason when told that he had died. They had moved the bed into a single room away from the unit. Where she could hold him and grieve in private. All the catheters, drains, and pacing wires had to be left in place until the autopsy. Yet I wondered, how could she cuddle the lifeless infant with plastic in every orifice?

This is cardiac surgery. Another day at the office for me; the end of the world for her. I was drawn to her like a magnet but had to stay away. In an hour I was due back in the operating theater. Needing to be in top form for someone else's baby. Another mother who cared just as much. What a fucking job. Sleep-deprived, psychological wreck operating on tiny babies on the other side of the world. I called the adult ICU to inquire about the trauma patient. The man who had recklessly crashed his car and killed another driver. He was doing fine. They were going to try to wake him up and take him off the ventilator. There was a certain irony in that. I wished it were the other way around. Forbidden thoughts. Surgeons are supposed to be objective, not human.

I took my despair to the canteen, where I glimpsed the miserable pediatric resident devouring breakfast. My instinct was to avoid him. Yet it wasn't his fault. I was the one who had done the surgery and I regretted not staying up all night to see it through. When he saw me, I could tell he was bursting to tell me something.

He told me that the girl had disappeared from the room, taking the dead child with her. No one had seen or heard her take off, and she hadn't been seen since. "Shit." I didn't want to continue that conversation. I assumed she had taken off into the night. Like her flight from Yemen. Now carrying a lifeless bundle. By now she could be anywhere.

I heard the news as I was stitching the patch into the first ventricular septal defect. When the Saudi hospital staff turned up for work, they found her. Two bodies lay lifeless in a heap of rags at the bottom of the tower block. She had removed the drips and drains from the little body before leaping into oblivion. To catch up with him in heaven. Now they were together in the cool of the mortuary. Inseparable in death. Two hundred percent mortality for me.

Most would end this tragic tale with the mother's suicide; the discovery of the bodies at the foot of the tower block. A devastating end to two fragile lives. But real-life heart surgery is not a soap opera. The job goes on. There were too many unanswered questions. So I went in search of answers.

I always attend the autopsies of patients I operate on. First, to protect my own interest, to make sure the pathologist understands what has been done and why. Second, to see if anything could have been done better.

To spend all day, every day with the dead makes mortuary people different, as I knew from my time at Scunthorpe War Memorial Hospital. The technicians work like butchers. Slicing open the carcass. Removing the entrails. Sawing off the cranium to lift out the brain. Here, an aging Scottish pathologist ruled the roost. Resplendent in green plastic apron and white Wellington boots. Sleeves rolled up. Cigarette dangling from his mouth. He was grunting away to himself. Documenting the cause of death of the man killed by my trauma patient. Fractured neck and brain hemorrhage, together with ruptured aorta. High-speed crash injuries. I was new to him; surgeons didn't visit the mortuary very often. Mercenaries were rarely interested in learning from their failures.

That morning, seven naked corpses were lined up on separate marble slabs. My attention was immediately drawn to the mother and child. On tables side by side, so far untouched. I explained to the Scotsman that I was pressed for time. He was grumpy but cooperative as the technician joined him. Only the child was officially my patient. His head had hit the ground first. The skull was split open, with the brain shattered like a jellied aspic dropped onto the floor. There was little blood because he was already dead. I had an important question about the brain. Did the boy have tuberous sclerosis, the brain pathology that goes with rhabdomyomas in the heart? This condition causes fits and could have precipitated his death. Eventually the microscope told us that he did.

I reopened the chest incision myself. Unpicking the stitches. Was I correct about the disconnected pacing wire? It was difficult to know because the mother had pulled it off after death. But there was a clue. A blood clot squelched out from beside the right atrium. In every other respect, the surgery had been successful. The tumor had virtually gone, the obstruction relieved. The Scotsman dropped the heart into a jar of formaldehyde and kept it on the shelf as a rare specimen. Eager to maintain momentum, the technician sliced open the abdomen and eviscerated the child. All organs back to front, floating in heart failure fluid but otherwise normal. Cause of death: congenital heart diseases—operated. A second technician came along, placed the brain and guts back into the abdominal cavity, then crudely sewed him up. After repairing the split in the head, the boy was stuffed into a black plastic bag. End of story. Blood and body fluids washed from the marble slab. Not a trace left of his tragic short life. No one to bury him.

I was drawn to her black, broken body now naked on the next slab. So thin. Mercifully, her beautiful head and long neck were intact. Once sparkling eyes wide open, but now dimmed and fixed on the ceiling. Her injuries were obvious without slicing her open. Broken arms and legs horribly distorted. Swollen abdomen from liver trauma. No one survives such a fall. She knew it. How different all this could have been had the boy survived. The happiness she would have experienced watching him grow up with a heart that worked. I watched the technician fold the scalp over her face and remove the top of the skull with a circular saw. Lifting the lid on her tragic memories. Why did she never speak? Like an archaeological dig, the vital clues emerged. Above the left ear she had a healed skull fracture with damage to the dural membranes and brain beneath. This involved Broca's area, the zone of the cerebral cortex responsible for speech. When the Scotsman carved her soft brain into slices, the scar became more apparent. It extended deeply, slicing through the nerves that led to her tongue. Injuries she was lucky to survive during her abduction in Somalia. The reason she never spoke. Why she understood but couldn't respond.

I had seen enough. I didn't want to watch the rest, her life blood spilled out onto the mortuary slab. Didn't want to bear witness to her other traumas. She died from internal bleeding, but a fatal head injury would have been kinder. I remember thinking, it would have been better had she died in Somalia. Had she been spared the misery of her life in South Yemen.

With that I thanked the Scotsman for his cooperation and headed back to where I belonged. The operating theater. Hoping for a better day. Desperate to do some good.

six

The Man with Two Hearts

A successful cardiac surgeon is a man who, when asked to identify the three best surgeons in the world, has difficulty in naming the other two.

—Denton Cooley

A N EXTRAORDINARY TWIST OF FATE LED TO THE CHANCE encounter. I had traveled to San Antonio, Texas, for the 1995 congress of the US Society of Thoracic Surgery. It was there while wandering around the Alamo that an executive in the cardiovascular industry asked me to give an opinion on a new product. He took me back to a corporate meeting with an engineer whose name I was well familiar with: Robert Jarvik. The device under consideration was a small turbine pump designed to boost blood flow down the legs of patients with severe peripheral arterial disease. When the company men moved off to their dinner with clients, Jarvik turned to me and said, "Come up to my hotel room, I have something interesting to show you." I am always wary of such invitations from men, but on this occasion I was intrigued.

First, he filled the sink in the bathroom. Then he took out a small plastic container from his briefcase. Like a sandwich box. In the box was a thumb-size titanium cylinder with an attached vascular tube graft and silicone-covered electric power cable. He put the titanium cylinder in the water, attached the cable to a tele-phone-sized controller, and switched it on. Whoosh. This small continuous flow pump shifted around 5 liters of water in a minute, redirected through the graft back into the sink. Without noise or vibration.

Rob Jarvik's New York City–based company had been working on the concept of a left ventricular booster pump for some years. It was a revolutionary new type of artificial heart, designed to be "functional but forgettable" for the patient, and very different from his original total artificial heart, the Jarvik 7.

Then I said something stupid. "This is a great pump for water but if you put it into the bloodstream it will clot. Or chew up the red cells." As if Jarvik hadn't considered these issues. I quickly recovered and added, "But I would love to work with you to test it. Away from the Food and Drug Administration. If it looks good we could use it in the UK long before you will get permission over here." A punt in the dark. But Jarvik appeared amenable. He told me he was already working with a center in the United States, in Houston—the Texas Heart Institute, with Bud Frazier, the head of the transplant service. Frazier was America's foremost advocate of mechanical circulatory support devices. He asked, "Would you like to meet Dr. Frazier? He's at the meeting." So off we went to find him.

Bud was 100 percent Texan. Wearing Stetson and cowboy boots with a well-tailored suit. Both charming and understated, he was a collector of antiquarian books. He expressed confidence in the new pump, known at the time as the Jarvik 2000, the year 2000 being the projected date for human implants if the laboratory research work went well. He invited me to see the calves implanted with the pump at the Texas Heart Institute.

The Texas Heart animal laboratories were considerably more impressive than my human facilities back in the United Kingdom, filled with sophisticated modern equipment that I could never get for my patients. The calves were happily chewing hay in the stalls. The monitors showed the impeller to be spinning at 10,000 rpm, pumping around 6 liters of blood per minute. More than what was needed by a patient at rest.

Bud handed me a stethoscope so that I could listen to the faint continuous whine of the turbine in the bloodstream. I was wrong. It didn't damage the blood cells, and irrespective of the lack of blood-thinning therapy, it didn't clot, either. This was a revelation—potentially a monumental step forward for patients dying from heart failure. Right in front of my nose, with an opportunity to get involved. I returned to Oxford with an immense international project, through sheer luck. I felt as though I could fly back to London without the airplane.

As I landed, however, my euphoria likewise came crashing down as I contemplated the reality. I had no research funds. All I had was grim determination, the will to succeed. But within months I had raised sufficient funds from philanthropists to begin the research project. Now Cambridge had its pig-heart transplant program and Oxford had miniature artificial hearts. A veritable varsity match. Soon, in my new laboratory we confirmed what Houston had suspected. Continuous blood flow without pulse pressure was safe and effective. This changed the whole philosophy of blood-pump design, not to mention human circulatory physiology. It eliminated the need to replicate the pulsatile function of the normal human heart.

Against the background of this thriving research program, I felt justified in beginning a surgical heart-failure service in my Oxford hospital in 1996. There were many thousands of terminally ill heart-failure patients in Britain, but less than two hundred heart transplants each year. Those older than sixty years and most with deteriorating kidney and liver function were considered unsuitable for acceptance on a waiting list. Their lives would be terminated prematurely by increasing doses of narcotic drugs in the name of palliative care. My vision was that these desperately symptomatic patients should be helped by "lifetime" blood-pump support, an "off-the-shelf" mechanical solution that didn't need a dead person or frantic donor-heart retrieval by helicopter in the middle of the night. My megalomania told me to establish Oxford as a National Center for Mechanical Circulatory Support.

In Houston, Bud was already implanting a more conventional pulsatile ventricular assist device to keep patients alive until a scarce donor heart could be found. This was known as mechanical bridge to transplantation. Shaped like a round chocolate box, the Thermo Cardiosystems "HeartMate" pump was intended to replace the diseased left ventricle by filling and ejecting blood rhythmically. It was too large to fit in the chest, so it was implanted into a pocket in the abdominal wall. Out of this emerged a stiff electrical cable to the external batteries and controller. This "life line" also incorporated an air vent that hissed continuously in time with the pumping mechanism. Audible across the street. It happened that the average wait for a donor heart for patients with the HeartMate assist device was 245 days, though much longer for those with blood group O. This prolonged hospital confinement was massively expensive and psychologically damaging. With increasing experience, the Houston team gained confidence that patients should be released from the hospital. Not only that, but they thought that this reliable blood pump was ready to be used as an alternative to heart transplantation.

Frazier knew that the US Food and Drug Administration would not consider it at the time. He called me in Oxford. As we were working together on the Jarvik 2000, might we test the "Lifetime Support" concept with the HeartMate in National Health Service (NHS) patients? The Thermo Cardiosystems company would provide the pumps free of charge. This would offer a lifeline for the terminally ill patients who had already been turned down by the transplant centers, those who were breathless on minimal exertion, swollen with fluid, and housebound—the walking dead, though rarely walking.

This was the chance I had been waiting for. I flew to Houston to watch an implant and meet the transplant candidates who were living with the pump in the hospital. When asked whether I cared to assist with an operation, I jumped at the opportunity. The patient was a Midwestern college football player who had caught a virus. Virile to viral. Athlete to asthenic. The poor guy was wasted and waterlogged, his life ebbing away inexplicably. His girlfriend was at his bedside, not knowing what to say. What do you say to someone who needs an artificial heart? She was a long-legged blonde cheerleader who reminded me of my training in Alabama. Nothing to cheer about now. She had watched her boyfriend deteriorate, lose his place in the team, drop out of college. It took too long to realize that he was sick, that it wasn't drugs, as some had suspected. What should she do? Leave him and get back to her studies, or stick by the young man whose best chance would be a heart transplant? Life is a bitch sometimes. We seldom stop to think how it is on the other side.

In Houston, the OR nurses helped the surgeon into gown and gloves. They painted and draped the patient, leaving the whole chest and upper abdomen exposed. Once, this young man had rippled with biceps, pecs, abs, the lot. But now he was skin and bone, his distended liver bulging beneath the ribs. Heart failure is shit. The sanctimonious creeps who declined to fund our research in Oxford should stand here at the operating table. Frazier made the incision from neck down into the belly. The HeartMate pump needed a sizable pocket in the abdominal wall. When implanted, it looked like an alarm clock beneath the skin. This patient's heart was huge, all dilated left ventricle, which barely moved. While I was mourning the demise of this great athlete, Bud was concentrating on where to bring the electric drive line through the skin, searching out a position that didn't interfere with his belt and trousers, where he could keep it clean with as little motion as possible. He made a stab wound with the scalpel, and we hauled the line through. This was not a domestic electric light cord. It was more than a centimeter thick and stiff enough to prevent kinking of the air vent. It was his lifeline, as important as the fetal umbilical cord for now. Then we carefully stitched the pump outflow graft to the aorta as it leaves the heart. Obsessional stitching, otherwise it would bleed profusely under pressure. All that remained was to sew a restraining cuff to the apex of the heart and use a circular coring knife to make a dollar-sized hole for the pump inflow cannula. Now blood returning to the heart from the lungs would pass straight through the mitral valve and into the machine, his own damaged ventricle now redundant. But I was taken by the fact that Jarvik's new pump was barely larger than this inflow cannula. The titanium shell of the pulsatile HeartMate pumping chamber was huge in comparison.

Before activating the HeartMate pumping chamber, it must be filled with blood to expel air. Air in the brain, life down the drain. Poetic, but by then I was jet-lagged, sleep-deprived, and a touch manic. The technical team had made the connections. We were ready for the big switch-on. As the pusher plate mechanism started to shift in the pump housing, air hissed back and forth in the vent. Like a steam locomotive setting off. The chamber filled, then ejected blood into the aorta. Residual air fizzed and frothed through needle holes in the graft, gratefully making its exit. His own useless muscle was sucked down, no longer tense and quivering in an attempt to keep him alive. He had a new heart. Temporary, but I hoped it would serve him well.

I wondered how his girl would react to this pulsating, hissing monster inside him. Or the new appendage emerging from his belly. How long would she stay with him now? These were thoughts that I would never normally entertain, due to the lack of empathy that stems from continuous stress and fatigue. If I saw her again, I resolved to be kind. To tell her how well it had gone. That he would now get better and stronger. If he was lucky he could have someone else's heart.

It took a while to stop the bleeding. General oozing stems from the poorly functioning liver and bone marrow in heart-failure patients. Bleeding, excessive blood transfusion, then bad lungs and kidneys were a common scenario in heart-failure surgery. Now I needed to go to the airport for another twelve-hour flight. Back to a world where none of this would have happened. He would have been left to die. But I wanted to see the girl first. The young man's parents were with her. Anxious as hell together. As she looked up and recognized me, I told her quickly that the operation had gone well—a phrase that always triggers waves of relief. Five words that cut through the tension. Her sweet face lit up with joy, and she started to cry. So she really did care about him, not only that he had been a football star. I felt miserable for doubting that. His parents hugged and thanked me. *For what?* I thought. I just assisted Bud. But with good news, gratitude goes out to all. I wished them all the best and a donor heart soon. With all the misery that will bring for another family.

With the help of Professor Philip Poole-Wilson at the Royal Brompton Hospital, we soon identified potential candidates for the HeartMate pump. Sadly, the first and youngest died before we were given permission to help. The next seemed ideal. He was sixty-four, tall and slim. Already turned down for a transplant. Like the American football player, he had dilated cardiomyopathy, possibly genetically linked, more likely caused by a virus or autoimmune disease. An intelligent Jewish man, Abel Goodman had a huge heart and was virtually bedridden. Yet on the plus side, his coronary arteries were free from disease and he still had reasonable kidney and liver function. I hoped that would make the postoperative care less of a battle. And less expensive. His breathlessness was worsening, so he was propped up in the bed with pillows, unable to lie flat and with swollen legs and abdomen. Philip needed to admit him to the Brompton for medical stabilization, so I went to see him there. I always loved returning to that hospital. This time as my own man. More proper heart surgeon than music-hall joke.

Abel sat bolt upright in bed, with labored breathing. He showed sweat on his brow and the look in his eyes that says, "I'm not long for this earth." He was too distressed to talk. Too sick for a haircut, as we say. Ready to meet his maker, but secretly hoping his savior had come instead. I shook his limp hand. It was cold and slippery. Blood wasn't getting that far. I explained that the HeartMate pump would take away his terrible symptoms and that he was the first patient in the world to be offered this technology on a "lifetime" basis. Normally, it was reserved for transplant candidates. How long was a lifetime? I didn't know, but without it he would certainly die within weeks. At most. In my own mind, I thought he could go during the conversation. His head tipped back and his eyes rolled as he digested the information. Not much blood reaching the brain, either. Abel managed to raise his head from the pillow and murmured, "Let's get on with it then." I think he hoped it would be that day. Enough was enough.

It was 3:00 p.m. in London, six hours ahead of Houston. I called Bud to explain the tight time line. We would only be given permission to use the pump in a dying patient on "humanitarian grounds." We had one. Could we do it next week? The line went quiet for what seemed like minutes. Then one word: "Yep." I felt a surge of adrenaline and excitement. We would implant a mechanical heart at my Oxford hospital. I was an ambitious bastard. We all wanted to take risks. Not just for the patients, but for ourselves. Knowing that it would create headlines. And extreme animosity from the transplant lobby. Flying in the face of that curious attitude that it is better to let patients die than attempt something new.

The Houston team arrived at Oxford on October 22, 1996. That evening the anesthetists, perfusionists, and nursing teams gathered in the conference room. We needed to talk through the procedure and get acquainted with the equipment. Not to mention my Texas friends and their dress code. Cowboy boots and Oxford colleges rarely come together. Abel survived the transfer out of London. He was bemused by the cosmopolitan medical team but too breathless to care. The rabbi came to prepare him for death. The nurses told him he had a great surgical team and to think positive. And the ward orderly took his order for supper the next evening. He didn't want the ham.

Bud had never been to Oxford. With his interest in antiquarian books, I wanted to show him the Bodleian Library and the ancient colleges in the center of town. Different planet from Houston. We drank beer in the Eagle and Child tavern, where J. R. R. Tolkien and C. S. Lewis met regularly on Thursday evenings in the 1930s. I listened to his stories about being a helicopter medic in the middle of the Vietnam War. He would sit on his helmet to avoid getting his testicles blown off. Several of his surgical colleagues didn't make it. Bud kept his balls, and it showed. He had done more heart transplants than anyone else and more ventricular assist devices. He reminisced over the agony and the ecstasy of those days. Then I asked about the college football star. He was still wandering the corridors of the Texas Heart Institute. No longer in heart failure. Building up muscle again, but still no donor. His girl had gone back to college.

For me, this evening was the calm before the storm. As for Bud, he hoped it would be the beginning of a new era, where pumps would be used to treat patients with no other option. Why should they be inextricably linked to transplantation? It was a waste of life-saving technology. What other historic discussions had taken place in the Eagle and Child over the centuries, I wondered. This must have been the first about artificial hearts.

The morning was more relaxed than I expected. The pump company representatives sat chatting with Bud in the operating theater coffee room. His technical assistant, Tim Myers, was already helping the nurses lay out the equipment. They were excited but nervous, and not wanting to screw up in front of the distinguished visitors.

Abel came down from the ward with a procession of family and friends to see him off. Off to where was the question. He sat slumped forward on the trolley in a white gown. Head bowed, hands on his skinny knees, gasping for breath in anxiety. He just wanted to be put to sleep. When they passed me in the corridor, he raised his head tentatively and murmured, "See you later." The man remained optimistic to the last.

This time I would do the surgery with Bud assisting. My colleague David Taggart joined us as second assistant. For such a politically charged event, we managed to stay calm and businesslike. Almost to the point of levity. The pump's manufacturer realized that surgeons were not the brightest members of the medical profession. So they put arrows on the titanium pump housing to make sure we implanted it in the correct orientation. I appreciated the gigantic incision. Neck to umbilicus. I was never one for keyhole surgery. Although I was proud of my own abilities, I was embarrassed by our outdated equipment. The old saw juddered up the breastbone, almost failing to make it to the top. We made the pump pocket in the upper left abdominal wall. Then zipped open the tense pericardium to expose Abel's huge heart. Yellow fluid pulsed out over the drapes and down my gown. Like baptism. I worked through the implant process step by step. Doing it Bud's way. Pipes in for cardiopulmonary bypass. Go onto the heart-lung machine and empty Abel's heart. Carefully sew the restraining cuff to the apex of the left ventricle. And the vascular graft to the aorta. We cored out the disc of sick muscle from within the cuff and kept it for the microscope. Then in went the inflow cannula of the pump. Job done.

As in Houston, the critical last step was to remove all air from the system before the big switch-on. That taken care of, the titanium "chocolate box" sat securely in its pocket. Tim was told to "switch on." The noisy mechanism started up with the characteristic hissing noise and the final few bubbles fizzed out of the air needle. Abel had a powerful new left ventricle, one that you could hear across the street. But the patients get used to that. Like mechanical heart valve patients get used to the tick, tick, tick in the dead of night. It becomes part of bionic life and preferable to the alternative. Usually.

Abel woke quickly from the anesthetic. Perhaps too quickly. He was immediately taken off the ventilator and the tracheal tube taken out. I could tell that he felt different. He had a twinkle in his eye. And a cheeky grin. He had that relief and bewilderment that everyone has when they wake from an anesthetic. The "I am alive" moment. All four limbs moved normally. He had no neurological issues. I felt like calling the chief executive as Christiaan Barnard had done after his transplant. To say, "Sir, we have implanted an artificial heart and the patient is fine." But something told me to hold back. To remain cautious for a change. This wasn't about me. It was about getting Abel back on his feet again. I was worried that his blood pressure was too high. Far from his own feeble left ventricle, he now had a powerful machine driving the circulation. And he was pouring out his own adrenaline in response to the unknown. The intensive-care doctors needed to give him vasodilator drugs and sedate him for the night. And anticoagulation for his own heart's abnormal rhythm. I needed some sedation, too. The aftercare was as important as the surgery. Overall, it had been a great day.

No news is good news. I heard nothing overnight. Always on a tight schedule, Bud and the company men left for Heathrow early the next morning. I drove to the hospital at 7:00 a.m., filled with optimism and self-congratulation. Fantasizing about the headlines: "Oxford Surgeon Implants Artificial Heart" or "Dying Man Saved by Heroic Surgery." My smugness quickly vanished when I reached the bedside. I could see it in his face. That vacant look. He was drooling from the right side of his mouth and his eyelid drooped. He didn't greet me with enthusiasm and gratitude as I had hoped. He couldn't lift his right arm or leg. He had had a fucking stroke. Every possible expletive plowed through my cerebral cortex. The pump hissed at me. He was pink and warm with great blood flow but fucking paralyzed. After everything had gone so well. Why had no one warned me? Every instinct wanted to blame someone else. But for what? My gut feeling was that he had thrown off a blood clot. Either from his own heart or from the foreign surfaces of the pump or vascular graft. In which case we should give him the rapid-acting anticoagulant heparin, as the warfarin wouldn't have had time to take effect. But a neurologist colleague persuaded me to seek a head scan first. To document the extent of the brain damage and rule out a cerebral hemorrhage. If we gave heparin after a bleed into the brain, it would surely prove fatal. Whatever the cause, this was a catastrophe, not least of it the financial implications of prolonged intensive care. All to be paid for by my research funds.

I accompanied Abel to the scanner. Bud and his team were already at Gatwick Airport, unaware of the miserable development. I was too pissed off to call. Let them enjoy the flight back. I watched the scanner construct slices through the brain. The pathology was obvious but unexpected. Bleeding into the brain. Not only that. The bleeding originated from an area of previous stroke that was many months old. Definitely not recent. Why did we not know about that? It transpired that Abel's wife had no knowledge of it, either. He had headaches from time to time but had never suffered paralysis or weakness. Before now. It must have been a silent stroke. Now we had the "devil versus deep blue sea" conundrum. Damned if you do, damned if you don't. Abel was disabled but not going to die. It was either "think positive" or get out of the high-risk business altogether.

I flicked the switch. Abel needed cardiac and neuro-rehabilitation. Many stroke victims recovered with time and effort. He couldn't swallow, so we needed to feed him through a gastrostomy tube. The gastroenterologists inserted this directly into the stomach through the abdominal wall. He couldn't cough adequately, so he needed frequent chest physiotherapy. When he developed pneumonia, he had antibiotics. When he coughed so hard that he disrupted the skin around the drive line exit site, we revised it surgically. The physio-therapists worked hard to mobilize him. In three months, the paralysis abated to weakness. The weakness resolved with exercise. Soon Abel was on the move again. His speech returned. Swallowing improved. He restlessly wandered the hospital corridors. Rehabilitating himself. No longer breathless or swollen with fluid. No longer in heart failure. His life was returning. So was my determination to press on.

We always heard Abel before we saw him. The sound of the pump and the hissing of the air vent—like a snake but sixty times each minute. Not easy to live with, but better than breathlessness. One day I passed him sitting out of bed in a chair on the ward. He volunteered that he felt below par. When we persuaded him back into bed and attached him to the monitor, we saw the reason for that. His own heart was in ventricular fibrillation, that uncontrolled rhythm that is immediately fatal in an unsupported patient. Irrespective of the fact that the right ventricle was now functionless, the left ventricular assist device (LVAD) kept him going. Incredible, I thought. Yet this happened on five separate occasions. We defibrillated him each time. A quick sedative, apply the paddles and zap. His own heart started again. In time we noticed something else. His own heart was shrinking and contracting more vigorously. Replicating Bud's finding that the dilated cardiomyopathy heart gets better with rest. It was important to find out on a molecular basis why this happened. Could we stimulate the process of recovery with drugs or genes?

Had Abel died from stroke, our charitable support could have died with him. As it was, he survived and was rehabilitated. The HeartMate continued to work well, and we were close to discharging him from the hospital. Then the next patient was referred.

That patient was Ralph Lawrence. He had taken early retirement from his job as finance audit manager with the Rover car company. He and his wife, Jean, liked to dance. Folk dancing, barn dancing, ballroom dancing. Energetic stuff. And they enjoyed traveling around the country in their mobile home. Then, in his early sixties, Ralph found himself increasingly breathless. The chest X-ray showed a big heart, so the local hospital in Warwickshire referred him to the heart-failure clinic at the Royal Brompton Hospital, where Philip diagnosed dilated cardiomyopathy. The first step was treatment with heart-failure drugs. This was followed by a treatment that was new in those days—electrical cardiac resynchronization therapy with a special pacemaker. The aim was to better coordinate the contraction of different parts of the dilated heart, to make the whole heart more efficient. But the beneficial effects can wear off as the heart gets bigger. Now Ralph was in trouble again, severely symptomatic with a poor prognosis. Could he have a transplant? He was told, "No chance at your age." Strangely enough, Ralph accepted this. He agreed that scarce organs should go to younger people. He was a likable man with a supportive family, and we thought he would be an ideal candidate for the "lifetime" HeartMate.

Although unable to do anything, Ralph was stable. Not as sick as Abel Goodman had been. He had a few weeks to consider and reconsider the prospect. We gave the family the HeartMate patient guidelines to read—daunting literature even for those who could anticipate a transplant in time. No swimming or baths. Showers were fine as long as the electrical equipment was covered. Avoid tight clothing or dressings that might bend or kink the vent tube. Always have the emergency backup equipment available. If the yellow spanner lights up on the controller, it signifies malfunction. A red heart symbol with audio alert means loss of pump support; seek immediate assistance. This was all worrying stuff that Abel had had no time to consider.

I saw Ralph with Jean in my office at Oxford. They were not easily put off by the literature. By now life was intolerable. There were no more outings. He was sleeping propped up in a chair, ankles and feet too swollen for shoes. Likely to die suddenly at any time. And the family knew that. I was concerned that he was an insulin-dependent diabetic, but he managed that well. He was used to taking responsibility for his own health. He had a positive attitude and wished to proceed as quickly as possible. "So why not start today?" I said. I thought they should arrange to meet Abel to ask him how he felt about life with the "alien" inside him. I knew what the answer would be: "Better than heart failure. Better than being dead." Jean needed as much knowledge of the HeartMate as her husband. She might have to cope at home in an emergency. Perhaps even work it manually for him in a power outage.

We agreed on a date for surgery, a Wednesday just four weeks away. That left time to make arrangements with Houston, but this time there was one more consideration. The grapevine had generated widespread awareness of Abel's operation. Given the stroke, we had tried to stay low profile. But because we were planning Ralph's operation a month ahead, it was inevitable that information would be leaked to the press. This was a two-edged sword. Public awareness helped me to raise the money needed to maintain the program. Yet bad publicity in the event of the patient's death could kill us, too. These debilitated heart-failure patients were so far gone they would never be offered a hernia operation, let alone heart surgery. How to control the risk? Between us, we agreed that one newspaper should be given access to Ralph's operation to avoid a media scrum. First and foremost, the family needed peace when, or if, he should leave the hospital. The *Sunday Times Magazine* was the chosen route. The paper could have in-depth access to the whole undertaking as long as the patient and family were treated discreetly. In return we would be grateful if the *Sunday Times* would consider a charitable donation. Not payment. Without charity, Ralph would not get his operation.

The night before the operation, Ralph and Jean stayed together in a room provided by the hospital. Jean told the *Sunday Times*, "We were quite rested. He had come to terms with everything and was just happy that the operation was to go ahead." At 9:30 a.m.

on Wednesday morning, a sedated Lawrence took the trolley to
Theater 5. This time we set up a video link between the operating
theater and an auditorium. I was happy for the journalists and hospital managers to watch. In surgery we have a saying: "See one, do
one, teach one." I had seen one in Houston, done one in Oxford,
but was quite sure that I was not about to let anyone else do Ralph's
operation. Bud and I waited quietly in the coffee room while the
anesthetist put Ralph to sleep.

It was 5:00 in the small, stuffy waiting room. All day, every day,
it was 5:00 because the clock had stopped long ago. Only the stack
of empty polystyrene cups marked the slow passing of time. Jean sat
waiting for news, consumed by hand-wringing anxiety. At 2:00 p.m.,
the news came that she'd been waiting for. Ralph was being wheeled
back to the ICU.

On May 12, 1996, an X-ray of Ralph's chest and artificial heart
filled the whole front page of the *Sunday Times Magazine*. The caption
reads: "The man with two hearts—why a lump of titanium, polyes-
ter and plastic is ticking away inside Ralph Lawrence." It was a risk to
give a front-line national newspaper direct access to an artificial-heart
operation. Pictures in the operating theater, interviews with the family and staff. But they presented it well and now everyone could read
it. The prime minister, members of Parliament, even the queen. The
Sunday Times produced a pictorial blow-by-blow account of the operation, which helped us sustain the laboratory research program. We
had struck a chord with those who saw innovation as the duty of the
NHS. But not with the NHS itself. This technology cost money, and
there would be no support for it.

We always felt that it was Abel's high blood pressure that caused
the cerebral hemorrhage, so we kept Ralph profoundly unconscious
for several hours. It was the middle of the night when he regained
consciousness. Jean was sitting there by the bed, watching the visible
action of the pump thudding away in his belly amid the paraphernalia of intensive care. Through the oxygen mask, he said something

to Jean. "You're thirsty?" she queried. "No, is it Thursday?" came the reply. Two days later Ralph was out of bed, sitting in a chair. The next day, Saturday, he was walking around the ICU with the physiotherapist, whose job was to rehabilitate him.

Then, trouble. As I was jogging through Blenheim Park, the mobile rang. This time it was about Abel. He was in great pain and in hemorrhagic shock on the ward. He had suffered acute bleeding around the pump, which caused a huge swelling beneath the ribs. Just at a time when his own heart had virtually recovered. We had to get the pump out quickly and stop the bleeding. Otherwise he was going to die. I asked that they call in the operating team as quickly as possible.

I ran home faster than I should have done at my age and jumped in the car. The roads were quieter on the weekend. I was pessimistic that we could get him opened up in time. Either we would or we wouldn't. One had to remain sanguine. An agitated, overexcited, or anxious surgeon would never succeed in this predicament. I worked out what to do in the car. We could never reopen the chest quickly without causing damage. I would expose the artery and vein in the groin, cannulate both, and begin cardiopulmonary bypass. Then he would be safe. With enough transfused blood, we could maintain flow to his brain and switch off the HeartMate.

In the hospital, there was frenetic activity around Abel to keep him alive. The nurses and residents pushed his bed unceremoniously from ward to operating theater, scattering visitors in the corridors and elevator. Squeezing in units of blood from their soft plastic bags while the hematoma got bigger. In through one hole, out through another. Desperate stuff, like the movies. We managed just in time. Abel's blood pressure had fallen to half normal despite the transfusion.

I pulled the wires out of his sternum and ran the oscillating saw up the middle of the bone. As the edges parted, strips of shiny purple blood clot slithered through the gap. Bright-red blood spilled out from the lower end. I soon figured out that the change in Abel's heart size had altered the position of the HeartMate inflow cannula, that the rigid cannula had sheared open the apex of the smaller heart. This informed guess turned out to be correct. As I dissected open the inflammatory mass, I could see that the join between vascular graft and the aorta was secure. It was a straightforward decision. The pump had to come out. Either Abel's own heart would succeed in supporting the circulation, or he was dead. The easiest way to stop the inaccessible bleeding was to cool to 68°F. Then stop the circulation. In the meantime, I amputated the HeartMate power line and discarded it. The pump pocket in the abdominal wall was full of blood clot. We scooped it out. Making progress. *Great way to spend the weekend*, I thought.

This was a bitter blow for the family. Everyone was looking forward to having Abel home after five months in the hospital. While he was in good shape. The wives of Abel and Ralph were both waiting—one hoping for a miracle, the other now realizing that a successful implant didn't mean happy ever after. Bad news travels fast. The somber mood spread through the hospital. Abel's nurses and physiotherapists thought they had lost him.

For my part, I was surprised by the change in Abel's own heart. Months of rest thanks to the work of the HeartMate had reversed the disease process and changed his heart's globular shape back to normal. As we carefully dissected out the inflow cannula, we found the bleeding point, a tear in the heart muscle itself. I peeled off the crescent of muscle attached to the metal tube and kept it for pathological examination. Then we could compare it directly with the core of muscle excised to accommodate the inflow cannula during his first operation. This was better than rocket science. We would show that the enlarged heart muscle cells had reverted to normal size and structure. We could help sick hearts to recover. Were the structural changes sustainable? Would the hearts continue to function? We didn't know. Only time would tell, but it was a monumental finding.

The surgery took seven hours. We delivered the pump like a baby as I wanted to keep it. The inflow cannula site was repaired with deep Teflon-buttressed stitches. The heart looked like a dog's dinner, but it worked. It was contracting well, boosting Abel's circulation as we rewarmed the blood. We separated from cardiopulmonary bypass as if it had been a simple operation. There was bleeding from every cut surface, but the blood pressure was fine. Was this going to be the world's first successful "bridge to recovery" in a chronic dilated cardiomyopathy patient? The first time a machine had been used to cure a heart! What a week that would have been. The bleeding eventually abated, and we closed the chest and abdomen. A triumph in itself. Abel's family was ecstatic. Ralph and Jean were relieved. My staff was optimistic. But I was still unsettled. We were perched on a knife edge here. Yet I had no choice but to leave the postoperative care to the ICU team. I was exhausted at best. At worst? Psychopathic, I guess. Juggling too many balls in the air. Pushing my own life and other people's to extremes. Surgery I find easy, politics less so. And taking risks with open-ended bills from the NHS was stressful. More than individual lives were at risk here. Many self-interested but influential characters were claiming that mechanical hearts would never work. It was a battle to prove them wrong.

Abel remained stable for the next thirty hours. Everything normal. His kidneys were passing urine, despite the prolonged shock. For now, I was the hero, yet I was still uneasy. The stakes were too high. I was walking on water but waiting to sink.

I didn't have to wait long. Late at night Abel's own heart flipped into an uncontrolled rhythm called atrial fibrillation. With a rate so fast that the left ventricle was suffering. This is a straightforward problem that happens to almost half of heart-surgery patients. It should have been easy to fix, but it wasn't. None of the junior doctors on site dared shock him. So he deteriorated rapidly. I rushed into the hospital, but by then he was beyond help. Abel died with his family around the bed. I could do one of two things. Go ballistic and get fired. Or walk away. I did the right thing, passing Ralph's bed on the way out. Jean was asleep with her head on the sheets. Oblivious to everything. Ralph stared straight ahead. Replete with anxiety. His eyes followed me as I passed. He understood how I felt, and there was nothing I could say to reassure him. He had heard everything: "Shall we shock him? Should we call the consultant? What if? . . . " Then the inevitable.

There is such a narrow margin between life and death. Survival depends upon those present being able to treat the problem. On whether the correct treatment is applied and if it is done at the right time. Abel needed that electric shock to return his fast heart rhythm to normal. For that he needed someone with courage to take charge and rescue the situation. It didn't happen. I felt that he had died needlessly. After all that effort.

Thankfully, Ralph went from strength to strength, transformed by technology, learning to live with the "alien" inside. Pumping away noisily. Hissing through the air vent. Circulating 6 liters of blood each minute with a strong, bounding pulse. Within two weeks, he and Jean had both mastered the equipment. The most important aspect was dealing with the stiff white power cable as it emerged from his flank. It had to be kept scrupulously clean. The surrounding skin needed to bond with it, to integrate with the Dacron covering and keep the bugs out. Ralph's biggest risk was of drive-line infection, which was common with this device but worse for a diabetic like him. At the outset, diabetics had been excluded from consideration for this reason. Jean practiced dealing with unexpected problems. How to troubleshoot if the alarms went off, when life itself depended upon doing the right thing. She learned to pump the HeartMate manually, should the electric components fail. Then off they went, happy and confident, anticipating a new life. This was the speediest hospital discharge of any artificial-heart patient ever. Ralph came back for checkups every month. He and Jean were traveling again in the motor home. Making the most of his resurrection. He was happy.

The winter brought predictable problems. A cold. Coughs and sneezes. These caused shear stress at the stiff abdominal drive-line exit site. The delicate seal between skin cells and Dacron broke down. Bacteria infiltrated the break in the skin's defenses. Jean tried hard to keep the site clean. Normal drive-line care. Then it started to discharge pus, becoming hot, red, and sore. The general practitioner (GP)—he was under the care of the local family doctor by then—took a swab and started antibiotics. Infection made the diabetes more difficult to control, and higher blood sugar helped to feed the bacteria. After antibiotics for several weeks, a fungus intervened. We admitted Ralph to the hospital for a few days to try to get on top of the problem. By now there was an infected and painful crater around the line. We tried to revise it surgically. It certainly looked much better. And Ralph's own heart had improved considerably. He spent hours working out on an exercise bike. Building muscle. Fighting to survive.

Eventually the fungal infection reached the pump itself. I knew this was the writing on the wall. Bud was experiencing the same problem with his bridge-to-transplant patients, though none were diabetics. I called him regularly for advice. We knew we could never sterilize it with antibiotics. Could we risk removing it as we did for Abel? I was seriously contemplating that when the infection gained entry to his bloodstream. Septicemia, we call it. Now both the inside and outside of the pump were infected. The pig valves directing flow through the pump were covered in masses of fungus and began to disintegrate. There was no way out of this. I had to explain to Jean that it was too late for heroics. The septic shock had caused kidney and liver failure. Ralph was yellow now. His lungs filled with fluid as those valves in the pump started to leak torrentially. The Heart-Mate even sounded different. More like a washing machine as blood splashed to and fro though the pumping chamber, and its hiss more like a boiling kettle than a snake. For me, it was finished. Jean understood when I said it was inappropriate to try "Abel-type" heroics.

Ralph couldn't survive it. We should help his breathing with the ventilator and see him off with the dignity he deserved. He had helped to start something. As the *Sunday Times* presented him, "the man with two hearts" had done so well. Ralph died eighteen months after the implant, surrounded by his family. After all the suffering, they remained grateful for this chance at life and time well spent.

We learned a considerable amount from Abel and Ralph. They were pioneers. The earliest patients to receive an artificial heart on a "lifetime basis." We accepted that the "lifetime" had been short, but all life is precious, as any cancer patient will tell you. What we needed were better blood pumps—and we were working on that.

Ah, nothing is too late, Till the tired heart shall cease to palpitate.

—Henry Wadsworth Longfellow

W HY DO PATIENTS DIE AFTER HEART SURGERY? IS IT because the surgeon makes a mistake, damaging the heart through a technical error? Has the surgeon operated on the wrong valve or coronary artery? Or let the patient bleed to death? Very rarely is it any of these. Usually it is because the patient was so sick beforehand that his or her survival was at risk even if the operation went well. As in any other profession, mistakes can and do happen; but the majority die because the diseased heart gradually deteriorates metabolically during the operation. Complicated reconstructive surgery may take hours on the heart-lung machine.

The heart suffers during the period when it is deliberately stopped from beating by taking away its blood supply. That's irrespective of the protective solutions we infuse, none of which are perfect. At the end of the operation, the heart is just too weakened to sustain the circulation, tired yet potentially recoverable. When the bypass machine is turned down, the heart won't take over. Without help, the patient dies on the operating table. More frequently, it limps off the machine but gradually fails over the next few hours. We can flog it with drugs, but the die is cast in the operating theater. The longer the heart muscle is deprived of blood flow, the more likely it is to happen. Then off to the mortuary. Unhappy family.

I felt that this pathway to death was preventable. The heart just needed time to recover. Staying longer on cardiopulmonary bypass was not the answer. It made things worse. Longer blood on foreign surface interaction meant more whole-body inflammation, in turn causing worse organ function and more bleeding. As a young research fellow with the great Dr. Kirklin in Birmingham, Alabama, I was the one who defined the chemical and biological mechanisms of these damaging effects. So I was motivated to find a solution. Not only that. Our discovery in the early 1980s made the heart-lung machine safer and saved countless lives. A great start to my surgical career.

What about some other type of pump? A simple circuit without the complex oxygenator might work better. This could be used for a few hours, perhaps days, or in the worst cases for several weeks. Until the heart's own contractile function and the benefits of the surgical repair would allow the circulation to be free-standing again.

A safe and reliable temporary blood pump would probably save one-half to two-thirds of those who otherwise die. How do we know? Postmortem examination shows us that the heart is structurally sound in most cases. It just got tired. Give it a rest and support the rest of the organs, then the patient might get better.

Most pioneers working on pumps thought that they would need to generate a pulse to replicate human circulation. So early pumps had to empty and fill and be large enough to mimic the normal heart. Usually it was just the left ventricle that needed help. If necessary, separate systems could be used to support both left and right ventricles. But the early pulsatile devices with bellows and valves created turbulence, friction, and heat, resulting in an environment that promoted blood-clot formation and the disastrous complication of stroke—always a dismal and feared end point in the battle to save life.

At Allegheny General Hospital in Pittsburgh, Pennsylvania, George Magovern, the chief of surgery, was less convinced about the need for pulsatility. He argued that when blood reaches the tissues, it is through tiny capillaries one cell thick. There is no pulse in this micro-environment. Pulse pressure has already dissipated in the small arteries before reaching the capillaries. Should pulse be unnecessary as we had suggested, then smaller, less traumatic pumps could be made. Pumps that spin at high speed. and deliver between 5 and 10 liters of blood per minute. The pump just needed to be kind to the blood. So Magovern engaged his friend Professor Richard Clark, head of cardiac surgery research at the National Institutes of Health in Washington, DC, to work with him on the project.

It took the team five years to produce a spinning blood pump the size of a bicycle bell, weighing just half a pound. Electromagnets drove one single moving part—a six-bladed turbine. First called the AB-180, it was intended to support the circulation for up to six months. Long enough for bridge to transplant. It was so simple that one of the technicians attached a prototype pump to his garden hose and drained his fish pond with it. It performed well on the laboratory bench without damaging the red blood cells. Then it worked fine in the circulation of sheep. As a result, the US Food and Drug Administration sanctioned a human trial with the AB-180 in 1997, on the strict understanding that the pump was only used on a "last-resort" basis. A trial of pump versus certain death.

In February 1998, I was invited to Washington for a heart conference by the Food and Drug Administration to discuss the recent operations I had performed on Abel and Ralph. It was in this setting that I met Richard Clark. He had been expected to retire but didn't want to cut the umbilical cord yet. Cardiac surgery was his life. Over dinner, he introduced me to the AB-180, which had the potential to salvage those who might otherwise die from low cardiac output syndrome, or cardiogenic shock as it is known. He asked whether I would take him on as a research fellow for a year. I was flattered and suggested that he bring the AB180 with him.

On August 7, 1998, Richard and his wife arrived at Oxford—from skyscrapers to the dreaming spires, from the world's best-funded health-care system to the National Health Service. A stark contrast. Up to that point the AB-180 had still not been used successfully in a patient. Three valiant attempts to rescue shock patients in Pittsburgh had all ended in death. There was a distinct possibility that the US clinical trial would be stopped.

August 9, 1998. 2:00 a.m. The phone wakes me. Strange, as I'm not on call that night. It was a cardiologist from the Middlesex Hospital in London. She was looking after Julie, a twenty-one-year-old girl from Surrey, a student teacher who was home for the summer with her parents. She had initially complained of flu-like symptoms. A viral illness. Within days she was exhausted, listless, and short of breath. Then sweating but cold. Not passing urine. Dying, in fact. The district general hospital recognized this and passed her rapidly on to the London teaching hospital. The ultrasound scan showed a poorly contracting heart. It was viral myocarditis, a viral illness like a cold, but when it involves the heart, it can be fatal. Inflammation and fluid accumulation had destroyed Julie's heart function. The cardiac output monitor confirmed poor blood flow throughout the body. Less than one-third of what it should be. A desperate situation for a vivacious young woman who had been normal the week before.

The cardiologist had admitted Julie to the cardiac ICU for what we call a balloon pump, a sausage-shaped latex balloon attached by a thick catheter to an external air compressor. The catheter is fed through the leg artery up into the aorta in the chest. It inflates when the heart relaxes. This raises the blood pressure and marginally reduces the amount of energy the heart needs to expend. But you have to have some pressure and flow for it to work. In Julie it was bloody useless, just obstructing the blood flow to her leg. The leg was already blue—pouring out lactic acid. At the time of the call, the highest blood pressure was 60 mm Hg. Half normal.

After the publicity about the artificial hearts, I was considered the "Last Chance Saloon." Could anything be done? Any technology that would help? The shocked parents and younger sister had already said their good-byes. They felt Julie had gone when she was anesthetized to be put on the ventilator. Conventionally, the ventilator and balloon pump were their final option. They had made no difference. As usual, the blood pressure dropped even further after the anesthetic drugs.

Most patients with viral myocarditis get over it. Like influenza, the effects of the virus dissipate and the heart recovers. This was not happening with Julie. The lethal blood chemistry and deteriorating organ function had gone too far. She was within the vicious cycle of acute heart failure that leads, inevitably, to death. In the middle of the night, you sometimes feel like saying, "Sorry I'm not on call. I've had a few beers. I can't help." I don't recall what I said that night. It was probably along the lines of, "Get her here as quickly as possible. I'll get the team ready."

Julie was brought by ambulance to Oxford as fast as they could manage. With doctors, nurses, and masses of equipment. I called Richard Clark, who rushed straight in to unpack the kit. Excited by the prospect of early action. My earnest Japanese fellow and right-hand man, Katsumata, came at top speed to assist.

We met Julie and her helpers in the Accident Department following a harrowing sixty-mile dash from London. By then Julie's liver and kidneys had failed and her blood pressure was negligible. We had no choice but to rush her straight into the operating theater. She was as good as dead. The parents hadn't yet arrived. They were struggling to get out of London even at that time in the morning.

One thing that subsequent media reports stated was incorrect. "Westaby had been given the green light from his hospital's ethics committee to use the AB-180." Wrong. No one but me had any idea that we had the device. And I had no insight into the fact that we might need it so quickly. Up to now, it had 100 percent mortality—statistically significant. But I was not the kind of doctor who would let a young patient die because of a bureaucratic detail.

It was fortunate that Brian, the perfusionist, had the heart-lung machine primed and ready. The intensive-care doctor accompanying Julie already thought that they were too late. When I put a hand on Julie's leg, I too suspected she was dead. It was white and cold and the veins looked empty. Her feet were blue. Even so, it was difficult to move her quickly. The drips, ventilator, and balloon pump had to be shifted carefully. She didn't weigh much. Katsumata and I lifted her gently onto the operating table. Sister Linda was scrubbed up, gowned and ready.

Dawn, the second nurse, stripped away Julie's white hospital robe. Her urinary catheter was caught in part of the equipment, stretched like a bungee cord, the inflated balloon still inside her bladder. Dawn fixed it. I told Linda to paint up with skin prep and get the drapes on. Katsumata and I scrubbed with haste. What was more important now? Survival or sterility? Dr. Mike Sinclair, our anesthetist, was grappling with the multiple lines and drugs, trying to make sense of it all and being helped by the visiting anesthetist, who held the key to the puzzle. It didn't matter what went into the lines. Nothing was helping. The Grim Reaper was perched on the operating light. I asked Mike to focus the beam on Julie's chest and grabbed the scalpel.

The blade went straight through, hard onto the bone. At one stroke. Forget the electrocautery. We didn't need it. By now there was no circulation. No bleeding from skin or fat, and Julie's heart rate was agonizingly slow. I ran the saw up the sternum. We wedged in the retractor and swiftly slit open the pericardium with scissors. Mike pointed out that the ECG was slowing to a stop. I didn't need him to tell me that. I was watching Julie's swollen, virus-ridden heart. Squirming in a pathetic sort of way. Like one of those toys where the battery is almost flat. The tin soldier beating his drum slower and slower till his arm finally stops in the air. Spent.

While the heart was stopping, I kept moving. I stitched purse-string sutures—running stitches that can later be pulled shut to close like a purse—in the aorta and the right atrium to hold the bypass tubes in place. The aorta was soft with no pressure, the right atrium tense to the bursting point. Every bite of the stitches pissed out dark-blue blood. It carried no oxygen, as there was barely any blood flow to her lungs. By now I wondered whether she was retrievable.

Working like clockwork and without words, we shoved in the cannulas to connect the bypass machine. Between each critical step I took the agonally flickering little ventricles into my fist and hand pumped—hard and rhythmically, like squeezing juice out of a grape-fruit. This internal cardiac massage was to maintain a semblance of blood flow to Julie's brain and coronary arteries. That's all that mattered. Forget the guts and offal. Just keep the brain and heart alive with whatever oxygen remained in the sticky blue blood.

Katsumata, a man of few words, murmured, "Don't mention the war." Wry Japanese humor used between us in times of stress. I told Brian to go onto bypass even before the venous drainage pipe was connected to the circuit. Almost black blood drained sluggishly into the tubing. In our haste, we had an air lock in the drainage pipe from the right atrium. No big deal. Lift the tubing. Air floats to the top. Drop it down onto the table and the air whizzes off into the reservoir. Now peace. The empty heart started to beat steadily now that it was receiving blood from the machine. Blood oxygen levels increased rapidly. The black blood turned red again. Lactic acid was filtered away. Julie was safe, as long as her brain was not damaged. A just-in-time job.

I turned to Richard. "How do we implant this thing?" It seemed straightforward enough. There was an inflow tube, which I felt to be unreasonably rigid. This would be inserted into the left atrium to drain well-oxygenated blood from the lungs into the centrifugal pump. The pump would become her new left ventricle. Then there was a vascular graft to return blood to the aorta, and then circulate it around the body. Simple. The device itself would sit in the right side of the chest between lung and heart. With the left side of the heart effectively bypassed, her brain and body would be safe. So let's get on with it.

Richard handed over the sterilized equipment to Linda. I wondered how best to insert the stiff inflow tube into the small, thin-walled chamber. The entry point had to stay blood tight for a long time. Instinctively, I thought we should sew a tube of human aorta to the left atrium. This would provide a degree of flexibility to the inflow cannula entry site and make it safer to remove without leaving a sizable hole in the heart itself. This simple trick could make the difference between success and failure. Life or death.

We kept a selection of donated human heart valves and bits of blood vessel in an operating theater fridge for emergencies. I had a special team whose job it was to arrange the donation from bereaved relatives and rescue the parts from the autopsy room. Human tissue proved invaluable for congenital heart surgery in which we have to rebuild children's hearts. Spare parts, pickled and preserved.

Dawn found a suitable tube of donor aorta in the fridge. In a sterile bottle. I carefully sewed this to the only accessible part of Julie's small left atrium and slid in the inflow cannula. A bit Rube Goldberg. Making it up as we went along. Then I sewed the outflow graft of the AB-180 to the aorta, using a side clamp. Careful blood-tight stitching. One last thing to do. The combined power cable and fluid-lubrication port needed to be passed out through a stab wound in the upper abdominal wall. It looked like we were wiring androids. I passed it to Richard. He connected it to the power supply.

By now, with steady blood flow from the bypass machine, Julie's own heart was beating again. But it was still feeble. I decided that we should support her for thirty minutes more before attempting to switch from cardiopulmonary bypass to the AB-180. Although the AB-180 would take over from the inflamed and swollen left ventricle, the right ventricle had to look after itself. With better blood flow, the cut tissues started to bleed. What's more, she had cooled as she was dying. With the heat exchanger in the bypass machine, her body temperature started to rise again.

I grew tired and a little impatient. I asked Mike to ventilate the lungs and Brian to leave some blood in the heart. We needed to fill Julie's own heart before switching on the AB-180. Otherwise the pump would suck the heart empty and obstruct. We needed to slide almost imperceptibly from one to the other. But how? I told Brian to stop the bypass machine altogether. He did, and this confirmed that Julie's own heart was useless. Then I told Richard to switch on the AB-180 and turn up the flow steadily to 5 liters per minute, equivalent to normal heart output.

An excited Richard flipped the switch and turned it on. Immediately, the pump came to life. Julie now had bright-red blood reliably coursing around her body. Simple plumbing, but joyous.

There was no blood pressure trace. No systole or diastole. Just flat-line continuous flow from the centrifugal blood pump. Would it work? Up until that point, there had been 100 percent mortality in humans. Sure enough, we would find out in the next few days.

But we could tell from the blood samples that it looked good. Julie had relatively normal biochemistry. What's more, the homograft tube worked well. There was no bleeding around that crazy stiff inflow tube. This had been a major problem in the three American patients. The turbine was spinning at 4,000 rpm, with a flow exceeding normal cardiac output. The pump itself was perched comfortably on Julie's right diaphragm. We had succeeded in keeping her alive.

Somewhat perturbed by the flat-line pressure trace, Mike asked Brian to switch the balloon pump on again. This produced a feeble pulse wave on the trace but no difference in blood flow to the body.

We soon confirmed that pulse wave was much less important than blood flow. Every cell of the body needs well-oxygenated blood, glucose, protein, fat, minerals, vitamins. But it didn't matter whether the blood had pulse or no pulse in it. Flow was the key. This was a major discovery at the time. Systole and diastole had always been considered vital in the human circulation. You had to measure them. If blood pressure was low, you had to get it up as a matter of urgency. But not with a continuous flow pump. Low blood pressure actually provided less resistance for the pump to work against. When pressure went up, pump flow went down. Counterintuitive physiology. We had to get used to it.

It was almost 8:00 a.m. The summer sun shone brightly on the dreaming spires. I left Katsumata to close the chest and went to warn the ICU about the impending arrival. Something different. For the next twelve hours, Julie's critical period, she would have no pulse. An average blood pressure of 70 mm Hg was fine. Her kidneys had quit. She would need dialysis for a few days. And she was a little yellow. The liver was suffering as well. By most criteria, she had been dead. But we hoped she would live now. Good or what?

Sister Desiree asked whether I had talked to the family. They were sitting in the relatives' room. Mom, Dad, and little sister. Totally exhausted after chasing around the south of England, awash with tea and sympathy but still expecting bad news. "Go and tell them what's going on," Sister ordered. "Celebrate later." At that point I was unsure about what I could tell them. Try this. "Your precious daughter arrived too late. We all thought she was dead despite the ventilator and balloon pump. But we implanted an unlicensed, previously unsuccessful machine from America. And now we have resurrected her from the dead. As long as her brain still works, that is!" That was the harsh truth of it all.

I walked into the miserable relatives' room. Clock still stuck on 5:00. Three heads bowed, hands wrung in laps. The heads looked up in synchrony. They didn't know who I was but suspected that I was there to tell them the worst. Then they could read my expression. With mask dangling down and blood on my theater shoes, I looked pleased. Not the sycophantic, forced look of sympathy that doctors use to give bad news. Julie was still alive. A miracle of technology. I didn't explain that it was new and untested technology that had never succeeded before. The nurse allocated to Julie's ICU bed slipped in behind me—quite appropriately, to hear what I would tell them. But nurses hate it when I suggest that everything will be fine. They want me to look grave and talk about a critical period. In case something goes wrong. They don't want me to put the unit under too much pressure. Pressure to get things right.

All I could tell the family was that the pump we had used was keeping her alive and we had been very lucky. It had only arrived from the United States two days before. We had only unpacked it when Julie was already on the heart-lung machine. "What are the chances now?" Julie's mother asked.

I told her that we hoped it would keep her alive until we could arrange a transplant. We weren't a transplant center, but I would talk to one and make it happen. It wasn't the time to mention that I was scheduled to be in Japan in three days' time.

I left the relatives and was told that Mike and Katsumata were bringing her around. Her mom and dad would be able to see her soon. It might be distressing for them. There were many tubes and lots of equipment attached to her diminutive body. But it would be better than visiting her on a slab in the morgue, with a sunken white face and waxy cold hands, lips bruised from the tracheal tube. I knew well from experience. Anything was better than that.

Sister Desiree was there to sort things out, to unravel the drips, plug in the machines, and calibrate the monitors. Get it all absolutely right. Desiree and Katsumata would be experts on the AB-180 by the end of the morning. For now they had to get used to looking after the girl with no pulse. This team didn't need me. That was just as well. My mobile phone rang. The message just discernible. The medical director wants you to come to the office.

I was expecting that. Medical directors are the Stasi—the secret police—from a hospital doctor's standpoint. Put simply, they are there to ensure that no one does anything new or interesting. Anything that might generate bad press for the hospital. The medical director's face was like thunder. How dare I use an unregulated device! Who knew about this? Was the ethics committee involved? What on earth was I doing trying to keep this young girl alive? He didn't say that, but that's how it came across. I didn't respond. Just sat there in my blood-stained theater gear. Thinking, *Get a life.* I said I didn't have time for this. Needed to get back to the patient. His parting comment: "If you do anything like this again, you'll be out." This reminded me of repeated threats to send me to "Bad Boys Boarding School" as a child. It never worked.

I went directly back to the ICU. Julie's family was now by the bedside. Desiree was explaining the paraphernalia keeping her afloat. Breathing machine, balloon pump driver, AB-180 console, infusion pumps, warming blanket. And they were bringing in the dialysis machine because her kidneys had quit. By now the operating theaters were waiting to start the day's planned cases. I told them I was ready. The first patient was a premature baby with a big hole in the heart. The parents were getting anxious. So forget the sleepless night. I was buzzing with caffeine and adrenaline.

Between operations I kept going back to Julie. I couldn't see the bed for doctors. One of my cardiology colleagues was trying to get good ultrasound pictures of Julie's heart without interference from the adjacent pump. These were causing great interest. The left ventricular muscle was completely offloaded. It was doing no work; well and truly rested. Only a slight twitch to show that electrical activity continued. The flat line on the monitor unnerved some of the medical staff.

By early evening, everything was stable. The crowds had dispersed. With an empty left ventricle and low blood pressure, the balloon pump was superfluous. Not only that, it was partly blocking the leg artery. Just another route for bacteria to gain entry to her system. I insisted they remove it. Katsumata lived in the hospital complex. Desiree a couple of streets away. They said they would keep a close eye, so I set off to get home for the night. Away from the madhouse.

By early morning, Julie was awake. With the breathing tube down her throat she was frightened and agitated. She had no idea of her whereabouts or why she had apparatus emerging from every orifice of her body. And clearly she was in pain. We needed to sedate her again. Just enough, though, because too much would drop the blood pressure. An injection of barbiturate into the drip, and she drifted away again. Into oblivion. The best place to be in these circumstances.

I put a stethoscope over the sternum. There was the loud continuous whirring sound of the magnetically suspended turbine. Still set at 4000 rpm and pumping 5 liters per minute, the volume pumped by a normal heart. Few at the bedside, on the ICU, in the hospital, in Oxford, or in the United Kingdom realized the significance of this single case. Pulseless flow was causing Julie's organs to recover. Brain, kidneys, then liver. Pioneers of artificial-heart technology had denied this was possible. What was the significance of this finding? Why was I starting to get excited? Because if non-pulsatile flow worked this well temporarily, then the new Jarvik Heart should be successful in the longer term.

At 7:00 a.m., I was summoned to the phone at the nurse's station. Somebody with an American accent wanted to speak to me. It was George Magovern, the man who had started the AB-180 project, calling from Pittsburgh. Well after midnight there. Richard had called him with the news, and he wanted to thank me personally. The engineering team was still out celebrating. They wished Julie luck, hoped we could keep her going till a donor heart became available. I said we would try. This was the boost I needed right then. Something to put the skeptics (and medical director) in perspective.

The next day, we took her off the ventilator and removed the tracheal tube. Miraculously, her brain seemed fine. She could talk to her parents. And there was more urine in the bag. I watched the flat line on the monitor screen. Then noticed something. She had changed her regular heart rhythm to irregular atrial fibrillation. Not unusual in itself. But when there was a long pause after irregular beats, a definite blip appeared on the arterial trace. When her own heart was allowed to fill for long enough, it was starting to eject blood. I wondered whether her heart was beginning to recover. Most cases of viral myocarditis recover with medical treatment before they ever reach the shock stage. So why would we want to transplant Julie if her own heart was getting better? It was simply the conventional treatment for severe heart failure. I suggested that we give her a dose of steroids to help decrease the swelling in the muscle. Witchcraft, but if nothing else it would make her feel better.

Now I had a difficult decision to make. It was Wednesday. Through some curious oversight, I was scheduled to talk at a conference in Japan on Friday and another in South Africa on Saturday. Unbelievable planning. The dates had been written in the diary as if it were London and Birmingham. But it was possible. The question was whether I should go at all. With the time differences, I had difficulty working out how long I would be away. But no one is indispensable. I had a great team. Julie was stable, so I decided to go.

Before I set off, we had a team meeting. Katsumata, Richard, Desiree, and the intensive-care doctors. We needed a careful plan for the time I would be away. The signs were good. Julie's kidneys and liver were already recovering. There were regular blips on the arterial pressure trace. Echo pictures showed improvements in heart muscle contractility. The plan was to keep her stable and let her recover slowly. Steady nerve. The pump was doing its job. So off I went to the airport, eager to relate the story to my overseas colleagues.

Less than forty-eight hours later, I received the sort of message I dread. When I switched on my mobile phone in Johannesburg Airport on Saturday there was a worrying text message from Katsumata. They thought Julie was bleeding into her stomach—a common stress response but made worse by anticoagulation for the pump. But. The big but. Her own heart was much better on the echo pictures. With the pump turned down, the left ventricle generated virtually normal blood pressure. I wondered whether the steroids had helped the heart but caused the gastric bleed. I needed to talk around the situation. I sent Katsumata a text saying, "Now in South Africa. Ring me." The call came soon afterward. I told Katsu, "Don't stop the anticoagulation yet. We can't afford to risk a stroke. Turn the pump down to 1,000 rpm for an hour. If the heart still performs well take the pump out." A long silence. I could sense Katsumata's "Oh shit" moment. Still silence until I said, "Come on Katsu, you and Richard can do it. Just get the bloody thing out."

Katsumata had called me from Oxford at 7:30 a.m. on Saturday morning. He went back to the bedside with Richard, and they called for another echo. Reducing the pump speed allowed the left ventricle to fill and eject more blood. Did Julie feel any different? They asked her and she told them she felt fine. She just wanted it out. There was no more breathlessness and still a normal blood-pressure trace on the screen. Richard knew that the lower the speed, the higher the risk of clotting in the pump or vascular graft. Desiree was starting a blood transfusion. She asked, "What did the boss say?" Katsumata responded with trepidation. "He said take the pump out and don't mention the war." And one last thing—"Only tell the medical director's office after it's out. We don't want him to have a stroke." "Then you had better tell the theater and get on with it," came Desiree's reply.

Richard and Katsumata explained this to Julie and her parents. The balance of risks. If her heart had already recovered but she bled to death from her stomach, it would be a disaster. Richard had been a chief of cardiac surgery in Washington, DC, for twenty years. Even he had butterflies. The stakes were high.

So, little more than a week after the implant, Katsu took Julie back to the operating theater. About the right time for a viral illness to get better. Richard didn't have hospital clearance to operate, so he could only watch. Had there been an issue, he would have dived in. There was no problem. Just cautious optimism at the prospect of success. Julie's heart was looking good. Stiffness and swelling gone. Blood pressure stable with a little help from drugs in the background. They still had a balloon pump in reserve, but she didn't need it. Katsumata washed out the whole chest with warm saline solution. Assiduously removing old blood clots from the chest cavity and from the pericardium surrounding the small but enthusiastic heart. He inserted clean chest drains, then closed the sternum with wire. Tight, and for the last time.

It was important to preserve the momentum. Julie woke up quickly and was much better off without the breathing machine. Now her own adrenaline pushed up the blood pressure; pulsatile again. The tracheal tube was removed later that evening. Desiree ignored her shifts and stayed with her. Encouraging Julie to breathe deeply and cough, despite the pain. The anticoagulation was stopped. The blood loss from superficial stomach erosions stopped soon afterward. We had done it. We had saved Julie's heart. When Katsumata called me, I had given my talk at a lodge in the Kruger Park and was already back at Johannesburg Airport. Headed home. Relieved by the news and in the mood to celebrate. Then Richard called George Magovern and his team in Pittsburgh. Spreading the joy. But none were happier than Julie's family, their grief and desolation lifted. No funeral. One day soon they would take her home. And Oxford only a grim memory.

In the 1990s, any patient who received a left ventricular assist device in the United States was committed by law to a cardiac transplant. Few other countries had access to circulatory-assist technology.

What we achieved with Julie became known as "bridge to recovery." In contrast to "bridge to transplant." It had not been done before in the United Kingdom. Bridge to myocardial recovery—the "keep your own heart strategy" soon emerged as the preferred approach for critically ill viral myocarditis patients. I was proud of that.

Just before Christmas 1998, the Pittsburgh engineers and researchers who had worked on the AB-180 filed into a conference room for a special party, arranged by Dr. Magovern. No one knew why—until Julie walked in with her sister. "The girl without a pulse" was instantly recognized from photographs pinned to bulletin boards. A face destined to grace the front pages. There was a moment of stunned silence, then loud cheers. Julie blushed as George shook her hand. "You being here is the best Christmas present any of us could have," he said. He was right. The company survived and thrived. The AB-180 was modified so it could be used without opening the chest. Now called the "Tandem Heart," it is used worldwide to support patients with shock in the cardiac catheter laboratory.

Julie remains well almost twenty years later. She works in a hospital. I look forward to a reassuring card from the family every Christmas. What's more, the medical director and I are still friends. Long may it last.

eight The Black Banana

Never surrender.

—Winston Churchill

Monday, February 15, 1999, 3:45 a.m. No one calls with good news at night. I had been in Sydney, Australia, for only thirteen hours after a twenty-hour flight. In pitch darkness, I scrambled across my hotel bed and knocked the receiver to the floor. The call was lost. I swiftly slipped back into sleep, courtesy of melatonin tablets and the bottle of Merlot I had drunk at dinner. Ten minutes later, the phone rings again. This time I am successful but irritated. What I hear is:

"Westaby, this is Archer. Where are you?"

Nick Archer was my excellent pediatric cardiologist colleague at Oxford.

"Nick, you know I am in Australia. It's the middle of the fucking night—what's the problem?" I didn't want to hear the answer. Nick didn't want to hear the cursing!

"Steve, I'm sorry but we need you to come back. We have a sick baby with ALCAPA. The parents know you and want you to do the surgery."

Oh joy.

"When?"

"As soon as possible. She has bad heart failure and is as good as we can make her. The ventricle is poor." Already there was no point in further discussion. I pictured the frantic parents. Desperate for an operation before it was too late. And four grandparents huddled around the bed. Trying to lend support but transmitting anxiety. There was no justifiable alternative. "Okay, I'll fly back today. You tell the team we'll do it tomorrow, whenever that is."

In the Southern Hemisphere, it was the height of summer. Early morning light began to penetrate the drapes. Further attempts to sleep were pointless. I stepped through the curtains onto the balcony, overlooking arguably the finest city vista in the world. Across Sydney harbor, the first hint of sunrise cast ghostly shadows over the Opera House. Flags fluttered on the masts in the harbor below. To the right, the tall white city lights stood out against the pink morning sky. The peace was broken by the shifting gears of a Harley Davidson. Maybe a surgeon racing to the hospital.

In Oxford, a real-life tragedy was unfolding for this little family. Kirsty was a beautiful six-month-old baby girl in whom fate had installed a lethal self-destruct mechanism—a miserable detail destined to end her life before her first birthday. ALCAPA is the acronym for anomalous left coronary artery from the pulmonary artery, which is an isolated and exceptionally rare congenital anomaly in the overall complexity of human anatomy.

Simply put, it's bad wiring. Both coronary arteries should arise from the aorta and supply the heart muscle with well-oxygenated blood under high pressure. They shouldn't attach to the pulmonary artery, as this has both low pressure and poor oxygen content. Early survival with ALCAPA therefore depends on the development of new "collateral" blood vessels between the normal right coronary artery and the misplaced left coronary. Eventually, these become insufficient to sustain blood flow to the main pumping chamber. Muscle cells deprived of oxygen die and are replaced by scar. In effect, the baby suffers repeated painful heart attacks. The scar stretches, so the left ventricle dilates. Then the heart progressively fails. The lungs become congested with blood, causing breathlessness and exhaustion, even during feeding. By six months, Kirsty already had the same problem as my grandfather at fifty-eight—end-stage heart failure, this time through a coronary anomaly. But because ALCAPA is so rare, the diagnosis is seldom made until the infant is terminally ill. Either then, or after it's too late. Kirsty's story was particularly harrowing. Fortunately, her parents were intelligent, had recognized that there was a serious problem, and were persistent in finding help for her.

Kirsty's mother, Becky, already had a three-year-old son. She was experienced and responsible and had contracted no illnesses, smoked no cigarettes, or drunk any alcohol during pregnancy. She risked nothing that could potentially harm the fetus inside her. All antenatal checks and ultrasound scans appeared normal. Kirsty was born on August 21, 1998, by elective Caesarean section with a spinal anesthetic. At first all seemed well, but not for long.

In the womb, the pressures and oxygen content of the aorta and pulmonary artery are the same, so Kirsty's tiny heart was safe. After birth, the circulations to the body and newly expanded lungs separate. Both pressure and oxygen content in the pulmonary artery fall. So, in infants with ALCAPA, both blood flow and oxygen content in that critically important left coronary artery fall precipitously, too. Even during the first attempt to breastfeed in the hospital, Kirsty was grunting. Becky noticed beads of sweat trickling from the bridge of her nose. Repeatedly, the effort of feeding made her fractious and distressed. This was distinctly different from her son. Becky asked for a pediatrician to review Kirsty but was told there was nothing to worry about. This is what fretting parents want to hear, but the truth was that no one had bothered to find out. Too much trouble. Piss-poor medicine. So Becky took her irritable but precious little bundle home.

Within weeks, Becky was certain that there was something seriously wrong. During every feed there was sweating and vomiting. Kirsty struggled for breath, clenched her little fists, and screamed till red in the face. There were many visits to the GP—as many as three times per week—and always ending in noncommittal, uniform reassurance. But they were tense, unpleasant encounters, as Becky was deemed neurotic and unable to cope. Despite Kirsty's rapid breathing, she had no fever. Chest infections were ruled out. Her belly was soft with no signs of stomach or intestinal blockage. All of the common pediatric problems were excluded. Family and friends offered rational explanations. It must be colic and would get better. But with her husband, Wayne, working in America, Becky became more and more anxious. Kirsty wasn't gaining weight. She had a pasty, washed-out look and a cough like the bark of a dog.

In reality, this baby was suffering repeated small heart attacks with excruciating chest pain that she could neither communicate nor understand. The human body can be outlandishly cruel.

Eventually, after the latest meltdown in the GP's office, Becky insisted that Kirsty should be referred to the local hospital. Twice she had chest X-rays, only to be diagnosed with bronchiolitis (inflamed breathing tubes) on both occasions. Then one day during her afternoon nap, Kirsty turned a terrible slate-gray color. She was barely responsive and limp. In panic, Becky snatched her up and rushed once more to the GP's office. But by the time they reached the receptionist, the baby was awake and pink again. There followed another put-down. Becky was told to stop fussing. That there were children to be seen who were actually sick. On this occasion, mother and child were acrimoniously dispatched with yet another prescription for antibiotics. Kirsty's huge heart was not detected.

Becky's frustration turned to desperation. Every instinct told her that if she didn't push further, something dreadful was going to happen. So she drove directly to the Accident and Emergency Department of the small local hospital. They were seen by a sympathetic female doctor who had children of her own. Recognizing that a mother's instinct was usually correct, she referred them on immediately to a larger city hospital for review by the on-call pediatrician.

It was a bitterly cold night, and they were left sitting in an unheated hospital corridor for several hours. Becky frantically struggled to keep Kirsty warm, but she became progressively more limp and gray. It was late at night when they were eventually seen. The first junior doctor suggested bronchiolitis and intended to dismiss them without investigation. Bronchiolitis seemed to be the only pediatric diagnosis these doctors had heard of. Becky was angry and frustrated, yet afraid that she would be thrown out if she protested. When she refused to leave without another chest X-ray, she was chastised for her unreasonable attitude. How unfair to inconvenience the hard-pressed duty radiographer at that time of night! So the sad pair were dispatched unescorted down poorly lit corridors and icy outside walkways to find their own way to the X-ray Department. Well beyond midnight, they returned, clutching the telltale picture. Becky presented it to a nurse, and they were parked once more.

Thirty minutes later, there came a dramatic shift in attitude from the hospital staff. Kirsty and Becky were ushered into a cubicle with different doctors. Now there were hushed voices and grave expressions and nurses bringing drips and drugs. That was even more frightening than being ignored. The previously mean, now sheepish nurse took Becky aside to explain that Kirsty was being transferred to the specialist children's heart unit in Oxford. By ambulance this time. Suddenly she was too sick to remain unsupervised. What did the X-ray show to trigger this frenzy of activity? Kirsty had an enormous heart.

Quite simply, no one had bothered to examine her properly. But it was now obvious on the X-ray film. When pressed about the previous X-rays at the same hospital, Becky was told that the heart shadow had been misinterpreted as fluid. Sorry, but it was an easy mistake to make. Some mistake! How do you describe anxiety that hits like an axe, drains blood from the throat, and takes your legs away?

When they arrived at the Oxford hospital, things were different. The pediatric cardiology resident met the ambulance and took them directly to the ward—a ward packed with children with serious heart problems. Beeping monitors. A hive of activity in the middle of the night.

Nick Archer arrived at 3:00 a.m. Examining Kirsty, he was immediately concerned by her body temperature. Despite Becky's best efforts, Kirsty was cold. She needed to be in an incubator and the diagnosis made as quickly as possible. An ECG and blood tests were done, then the echo machine brought to image the heart chambers. First it seemed like good news. All four chambers were there with no holes between them. But worryingly, the left atrium and ventricle were both enlarged, the ventricle dramatically so. This explained the heart failure and accounted for the striking chest X-ray appearances.

In little more than an hour, the cardiology team established that Kirsty had severe heart failure. Parts of the left ventricular wall now consisted of thin scar tissue interspersed with poorly contracting muscle. A rare finding in an infant but one that provided the likely diagnosis. One more test was needed. A cardiac catheter would confirm the coronary artery anomaly but would need a general anesthetic. She would have to be in much better condition before proceeding.

By now, Becky was overcome with grief. Physically and emotionally drained. Her husband was still away on business and she felt very much alone. Guilt and irrational thoughts frightened her. Had she exercised too much during pregnancy? Drunk too much coffee? Offended God? There has to be a reason for everything. Deep despair gripped her. Anxiety progressed to outright panic. She was certain she would lose Kirsty. As the winter sun broke the horizon, she lost consciousness for a couple of hours until the ward became busy, full of warmhearted people who tried to reassure her. Sure things were difficult, but there was a great team caring for Kirsty.

It was a full five weeks before she was considered fit enough for the cardiac catheter. By then Becky had Wayne back to share the pain. The evening before the procedure, Mike, the anesthetist, came to chat about the risks. Normally a jolly character, he didn't have much to smile about. He warned the family that Kirsty's heart was so severely damaged that they could lose her during the procedure. It was only fair to inform them. That night Kirsty was christened in her little bed by the hospital chaplain. Doctors, nurses, and other families gathered around the bed to support them.

Everyone suspected what the catheter would show. In reality, there was only one rare condition that did this to a baby—ALCAPA. Becky overheard the phrase "early surgery" and hoped that didn't mean a transplant. The parents stayed by Kirsty's bed the whole night, terrified she might slip away. In the morning, without sleep and paralyzed with fear, Becky dressed the baby in her best pajamas. Then tied a bow in her hair to go to the catheter laboratory. Ironically, it was Valentine's Day. As Becky put it to me later on, "A girl has to look her best even when she is poorly."

And of course, Dr. Archer was shown to be correct. They identified the anomalous coronary artery and set about bringing me home. Once I got on the flight, I started to sketch the anatomy of Kirsty's aorta, pulmonary artery, and abnormal left coronary artery. I knew that existing operations for ALCAPA had limitations, and a substantial failure rate. I would use the time on the airplane to work out an alternative. By the time we were drifting over Java, I had designed my new operation. Last on, I was first off the plane back in London. As I waited for the air bridge and the doors to open, the cabin services director handed me a bottle of champagne, wished me luck, and whispered, "You operated on my sister's baby." Small world. I thanked her. As the doors opened, a cold wind and a blast of reality hit me.

I called my colleague Katsumata and asked him to bring Kirsty's parents to my office with a consent form and the cardiac catheter on disc to show me. Kirsty needed surgery as soon as possible.

Becky looked tired and drawn when I saw her. She knew instinctively who I was. Her face lit up as they entered my office in a miserable cold modular building outside the main hospital. "We are pleased to see you," she said. "How was the trip?"

"Good. Restful," I lied. "We need to get on with this, don't we?" Katsumata managed to steal an electric convection heater from an adjacent office, and we broke the ice. They explained that a family member was a representative for a heart-valve company and knew me well. He had been expecting to see me at the meeting in Australia. They were sorry for my aborted trip but so grateful that I had come back. They wouldn't let anyone else touch their little girl. Despite the warmth, Becky was now trembling uncontrollably. With abject fear, poor kid. Finally, after weeks in the hospital the time had come. The day she might lose her baby.

I don't do transmitted anxiety if I can help it. It's more difficult for my anesthetic colleagues, who have to deal with the agonizing separation. I described my planned operation and explained why I felt it would be an improvement on existing techniques. The new left coronary artery would be constructed with a flap of aortic wall that would sit below a corresponding pulmonary artery flap to make a tube. The latter contained the misplaced origin of the left coronary artery at its apex. The product would be a new coronary artery that would be delivering high-pressure, well-oxygenated blood directly from the aorta—where it should have come from in the first place. Blood fully saturated with oxygen would then supply the failing heart muscle and prevent more heart attacks. Katsumata was intrigued and excited by this proposal. So much so that he rushed off to call the hospital's film crew.

With severe heart failure, the risks of the operation were substantial. Becky's shaky hand signed the consent form, and then I walked back with them to the children's ward. When we reached the bed, I was shocked. Kirsty's heart failure was the worst I had ever seen in any child. She had virtually no body fat. Her heaving ribs and rapid breathing reflected the congested lungs. Her abdomen was swollen with fluid. But she was still a pretty baby. Without urgent surgery, she would be dead within days. A voice in my head screamed, *Oh shit.* My mouth said, "I think we should make a start." I quickly walked away to the operating theater, not wishing to convey my concerns.

The anesthetists and the nurses were busily preparing drugs and catheters in the anesthetic room. Mike knew the score, having already anesthetized Kirsty for the cardiac catheterization. Some of the monitoring lines were still in place. "Do you really think you can get this baby through?" he asked. I didn't answer. I bid a good morning to the nurses and perfusion team in the operating theater, then went to the coffee room. I wanted to avoid watching Becky leave her baby with strangers. That is always an excruciating event.

When I returned, Kirsty was already on the operating table, covered in green drapes held in place with an adherent plastic drape. Just her bony little chest and swollen abdomen were visible. Now I could focus. Heart surgery needs to be an impersonal, technical exercise.

I joined Katsumata and my 6'-6" Australian fellow Matthew at the scrub sink. Only hours before, I had been at his hospital before flying back from Sydney. While we scrubbed in silence, the film camera was positioned next to the operating lights. There was a palpable buzz of excitement. We were about to do something new, rare, and risky.

There was no bleeding as I drew the scalpel blade along the skin over the breast-bone. In shock, the skin capillaries had shut down to divert blood to vital organs. Next, the electrocautery cut through the thin layer of fat onto the bone. This has a characteristic buzzing noise with a whiff of burning as the current cauterizes oozing blood vessels. This time there were few.

We cut through the sternum, then used a small metal retractor to crank open the tiny chest, bending and stretching the joints between the ribs and the spinal column. While we made our way down the layers, the other members of the team worked silently. The anesthetist administered Heparin to stop Kirsty's blood from clotting in the heart-lung machine. The perfusion team had set up the complex array of tubing, pumps, and oxygenating equipment that would keep Kirsty's body alive when her heart was stopped. Our scrub nurse was concentrating on having the surgical instruments ready to slap into my palm. During my work, I rarely have to ask for anything. This complex, highly coordinated work relies heavily on team consistency. Most have been with me for years, and I have great confidence in all of them.

As we pulled up the edges of the pericardial membrane to display the heart, Katsumata involuntarily uttered, "Oh shit." Back from his first cigarette, Mike popped his head over the drapes. I agreed that things were even worse than we had expected. Others could see on the video screen.

What should have been a walnut-sized heart was the size of a lemon. The dominant right coronary artery had many enlarged branches crossing over toward the left ventricle. While the right side of the heart pumped vigorously against raised pressure in the lungs, the left ventricle was hugely dilated and barely moved. Patches of newly necrotic muscle merged with areas of white fibrous scar tissue. All of this the result of the many small painful heart attacks Kirsty endured during her first six months of life. Katsumata was right to be concerned, but I didn't respond to his anxieties. We were committed to improving that blood supply and giving Kirsty a chance at life. She had survived to this point. It was our job to keep it that way.

Having exposed this heart, I began to question the wisdom of attempting this complex operation straight off a daylong flight. Yet what would have been gained by turning her down for surgery? Or procrastinating further. For Kirsty, there was no alternative. Urgent heart transplants were virtually impossible in babies. Re-plumbing of the heart's blood supply was her only hope. I was committed. No turning back.

The tiny pipes were inserted to connect her to the heart-lung machine. I gave the signal to go on. The perfusion technician turned on the roller pump and the heart gradually emptied. Technology took over, diverting blood away from the lungs and into the synthetic oxygenator. With the empty heart still beating, I cut through the pulmonary artery above the origin of the anomalous coronary. There was the opening of the vessel, like the pearl in an oyster. Now we had to connect it without tension to the high-pressure aorta 1.5 centimeters away. Simply trying to stretch and reimplant the origin of the vessel into the side of the aorta could result in thrombosis and blockage. So I pressed on with my new technique.

The delicate technical exercise could only be achieved by clamping the aorta and temporarily stopping all blood flow to the heart. We would protect the muscle by infusing cardioplegia fluid directly into both coronary arteries. The blood would then by flushed out and the ventricle would collapse like a punctured football. This induced state of inactivity is used for most heart surgery. It is reversed simply by removing the clamp on the aorta, which allows blood from the heart-lung machine to flow back into the coronary arteries.

For the reconstruction of this tiny vessel, the stitching had to be precise, accurate, and water-tight. The procedure went well. Just thirty minutes after the heart had been stopped, the conjoined flaps restored Kirsty's coronary artery anatomy to what it should have been. As the clamp was removed, bright-red oxygenated blood, rather than deoxygenated blue blood, flooded the left ventricular muscle. The heart changed from a pale pink to deep purple, then almost black in parts. Before reconstructing the pulmonary artery, we made certain there was no bleeding from the lines of stitching behind it. Soon the electrocardiogram showed incoordinate electrical activity, and the heart stiffened with renewed muscle tone.

Unusually for a child, the reperfused heart kept writhing and squirming in ventricular fibrillation. We used an electric shock directly through the muscle to restore normal rhythm. Ten joules—zap—the heart defibrillated and stopped wriggling. The heart was now motionless, but we expected normal rhythm to resume at any moment. It didn't. The purple ball fibrillated and squirmed again. The anesthetist's head popped over the drapes to request the obvious. "Shock it again." We did, and the same thing happened. It wasn't coming back.

There was serious electrical instability because of the scar tissue. We gave the appropriate drugs to stabilize the muscle-cell membranes. "Let's give it more reperfusion time," I told Mike. "Okay, I'll go out for a fag," he responded. Twenty minutes later, we tried again. Twenty joules—zap. This time her whole little body levitated from the operating table and the heart defibrillated. Although it slowly began to beat, it was barely more than a flicker. Ominous, but we had drugs in reserve to make it pump harder.

I asked the anesthetists to start an adrenaline infusion and told the perfusionist to cut back on pump flow to leave some blood in the heart. This was operating theater protocol. Like the military. You make a request to a medical colleague but give orders to the technical staff. If you give orders to anesthetists, they will tell you to piss off and do something different.

Mike and the perfusionist worked together to check and optimize the blood chemistry. My gaze was still fixed on Kirsty's pathetic little heart. The new coronary artery was fine. There was no kink in the tube and no bleeding. For the first time, the left ventricle was receiving well-oxygenated blood at the same pressure as the rest of the body. But it still looked like an overripe plum and was barely beating at all. Moreover, the mitral valve was leaking badly.

My mouth said, "Let's give it another half hour's support on the pump." What my brain said was, "We're stuffed. This heart has had it." Great operation—dead baby.

I didn't let the others know what I was thinking. This team had salvaged so many catastrophes that everyone expected me to pull it off. But I was starting to fade. I suggested that the cameraman should stop filming for a while because nothing was going to change. I told Katsumata to come to my side of the operating table while I took a break. I removed the gown and gloves and went to the phone in the anesthetic room. Mike followed. "Can you repair the mitral valve?" he asked. "Don't think so," was my reply. "I'll get Archer to warn the parents." I slumped on a stool and picked up the phone. One of the nurses put a coffee and doughnut in front of me. With an arm around my shoulder, she felt the cold sweat dripping down the middle of my back. "I will get you a dry top," she said.

I needed to focus. What, if anything, could I do to make things better? I was running out of ideas.

The left ventricle was scarred, dilated, and now globular—not the normal elliptical shape. This distortion pulls open the mitral valve and prevents it from closing. As the left ventricle tried to pump blood around the body, as much as half of it flowed backward to the lungs. Heart function is always temporarily worsened during surgery, but in Kirsty's case this had cut the umbilical cord between life and death. I had hoped that resting the heart on the bypass machine would help it to recover. It hadn't.

I went back, scrubbed up again, and switched with Katsumata. He said nothing but looked crestfallen. A clear message. I asked Mike to start ventilating the lungs and told the perfusionist to prepare to slowly ease off the machine. At this point Kirsty's heart had to take over and support the circulation. Otherwise she would die on the operating table. We all stared at the traces on the screen. Hoping to see the blood pressure rise. It briefly reached half normal but fell away rapidly as the pump was switched off. "Shall we go back on?" asked Katsumata. Watching the left ventricle flicker on the echo, the perfusionist questioned whether it was worth it. "She's had it, hasn't she?" was the message from behind the drapes. I wasn't yet ready to call it. Failure meant death for a little girl and lifelong torment for the parents

"Let's go back on, give it another half hour." This in itself was problematic. A long bypass time always lessened the chance of recovery.

The parents were waiting in the children's ward. Archer had gone to warn them. When we called him back, Becky insisted on coming to the doors of the operating theater complex with him. It's impossible to imagine how a mother feels in these circumstances. So I'll let Becky's own words, recorded in her diary at the time, speak for themselves.

> Dr. Archer sat us down. He explained that despite the best efforts of the surgical team, Kirsty's heart would not separate from the bypass machine. The surgeons were still trying but the prospects looked bleak. We may lose her. Then he had to leave. By now my head was spinning. I remember feeling sort of drunk. This wasn't the plan. If we waited patiently everything would be ok because that sort of thing only happens to other people.
>
> Then Dr. Archer came back. He told us he was so sorry. Every option had been exhausted. He would be arranging for us to go and hold her to say goodbye. I could not bear the thought that when I saw her again she would be cold. My baby was so soft and warm. Smelt delicious, hair like velvet, hot fuzzy cheeks. I just kept thinking that my heart would break if she was limp and cold. It sounds odd but it was such a strong feeling. Obviously this was our darkest moment. The thought of Kirsty fighting for her life and nothing we could do. We might as well have been on the other side of the world. My frenzied brain went into overdrive. If she died

they would put her on a cold slab in the mortuary. That hideously soulless place. If that happened I would stay with her until she was buried. I would fight anybody that tried to stop me. My baby girl would stay in my arms and God help anybody that tried to take her away from me. Those thoughts remain as clear in my head as they were on that day because I never felt so strongly about anything. We had made a really close bond with other parents on the ward. All day they had been popping in asking for news, praying for Kirsty and sharing in our hopes. When Dr. Archer left our room no one else came in. I didn't blame them. There was a horrible feeling of sadness. Everyone was so involved in each other's journey and now nobody knew what to say.

On the rare occasion that a child died on the operating table, I always talked to the parents myself. It was something I dreaded, the worst part of my job. The sliding doors to the theater complex opened automatically onto the hospital corridor. I was immediately confronted by eyes full of grief and desperation. I remember Becky said, "Please save my little girl." Poleaxed, I said nothing. Archer looked devastated. He had already done the difficult job.

I turned back to the somber theater, put on a new mask, and scrubbed up again. Mike had finished another cigarette. He said, "Things are no better. Can we turn the pump off?"

"No, I am going to try one more thing. Turn the lungs off. Run the camera again." This was my last-gasp attempt, something that could only be justified by the laws of physics and had never been done in a child. The tension on the wall of Kirsty's scarred left ventricle was elevated because of the size of the cavity. From a recent conference, I knew that a Brazilian surgeon had made a series of failing adult hearts smaller when a tropical infection, Chagas disease, weakened the muscle. The operation had been attempted for other types of heart failure patients in North America but was soon discredited and abandoned. In my view, this bold approach was Kirsty's last hope.

I was not going to risk stopping the heart again. I took a glistening new scalpel and cut the beating left ventricle wide open from apex to base. Like unzipping a sleeping bag. I began in an area of scar and carefully avoided the muscles that support the mitral valve. The filleted heart immediately fibrillated in response to cutting. This was fine, because there was no risk of it pumping air. Frankly, I was stunned by the unexpected appearance of the inner lining of the heart. It was covered in thick white scar tissue. To reduce the diameter of the ventricle, I cut away the tissue on either side of the incision until I reached bleeding muscle. One-third of the circumference of the chamber was removed. In an attempt to stop the mitral valve from leaking, I sewed the central point of its two leaflets together. This turned it from an oval to a double orifice structure like a pair of spectacles. Then I simply sewed the muscle edges together with a double row of stitches to close the heart. In the end it looked like a quivering black banana. A much smaller heart. Not for a moment did I think it would ever start again. Nor did my colleagues. Most of them thought I was crazy.

Word of the bizarre operation in Theater 5 soon spread. The curious gathered to watch, and the camera kept filming. We had to ensure that all air was removed from the heart, otherwise it could be ejected into the blood vessels of the brain and cause a stroke. After that, all that remained was to defibrillate and try to restore normal heart rhythm.

"We're done—try 20 joules"—zap—and the heart stopped quivering. For what seemed like an age, there was no spontaneous electrical activity. I poked the muscle with forceps and it contracted in response. This time there was a flicker on the blood pressure trace. Miraculously, the black banana had ejected blood into the aorta. Mike looked again at the echo. "It certainly looks different. Shall we try using the pacemaker?" I was already sewing the fine pacing wires into place. We arbitrarily set the pacing box rate at 100 beats per minute and switched it on. I told the perfusionist to cut back on the pump flow rate and leave blood in the heart. To see if it would eject consistently. It did. What's more, the echo showed that the mitral valve no longer leaked. At this point, I felt that we were in with a chance. Life really does depend upon physics and geometry.

It was after midday. By now Kirsty had been on the bypass machine for more than three hours. We needed to get her off it. Timed to perfection, Kirsty's own heart rhythm suddenly broke through the pacing. Coordinated natural heart rhythm is much more efficient than electrical pacing. It provided much better blood flow and pressure.

It was like pressing a light switch in the operating theater. Gloom changed to elation. My own adrenaline kicked in and my tiredness lifted. We gave Kirsty an infusion of adrenaline to help her heart take over from the bypass machine. Finally, I gave the instruction: "Come off slowly." We still expected the blood pressure to fade, yet the curiously reconfigured little heart kept on pumping.

"Off bypass. Don't believe it," said Mike. I said nothing. I looked over my mask at Katsumata, who murmured, "Don't mention the war." He knew that I had had enough by now. "Let me finish," he said.

"Sure."

I took a last disbelieving glance at the little black banana pumping away. I turned to the echo screen, where the incomprehensible flashes of white, blue, and yellow were also reassuring, like a blazing fire. We could see blood streaming through the newly constructed left coronary and a double jet entering the left ventricle through the mitral valve. A curiously reconfigured baby's heart that finally worked.

After the encounter at the operating theater door, both Archer and the parents believed that Kirsty had died. This was an unprecedented but awkward situation that I was too exhausted to deal with. I asked the anesthetic nurse to bleep Dr. Archer and tell him to come down yet again. "I'll get you a coffee," was her reply.

Katsumata made certain that there was no bleeding, then meticulously closed the chest. "Never been done before," he said, looking over at me. Soon afterward, Becky came down to the pediatric ICU in shock. She put her hand on Kirsty's little foot and exclaimed, "It's warm, it's never been warm." When she started to cry, I left. It had been a long day.

Dee, my endearing and eccentric secretary, drove me home to Bladon, some twenty minutes outside Oxford. I was restless with a mix of elation and fatigue. A huge red wintery sun was setting over Blenheim Palace. To wind down, I set out to run around the lake with Max, our German shepherd dog. Through the ancient oaks, we scattered rabbits and fortunate pheasants that had survived the shooting season. The shadows lengthened. Hissing swans told Max to piss off. The sun slipped away as I staggered by the water's edge. I left the park at the Bladon gate, crossing the road into the village churchyard. By St. Martin's church is Sir Winston Churchill's grave. Facing the tomb is a wooden seat donated by the World War II Polish Resistance Movement. And invariably, dead flowers with their heads dipped in reverence. Hot and gasping for breath, I sat to talk with the great man. Less than ten feet away in his box. Morbidly, I tried to visualize how his corpse looked now and considered how Kirsty should have been stiff and cold in the hospital mortuary. I had followed his advice. Never surrender.

Max irreverently cocked his leg on a neighboring tomb. Now I needed to sleep. I hoped that the phone would leave me in peace. It did. Kirsty survived.

The first time I showed the film of this operation was at a cardiology conference in San Diego. Edited down to ten minutes, the footage ended with a shot of Kirsty bouncing on Becky's knee just prior to going home. At this point, while I was still talking, the whole audience spontaneously stood and applauded. An uplifting experience. Like me, they knew Kirsty was a miracle.

We followed her carefully over the next ten years, watching the heart develop with echocardiography. She was a perfect little girl. Happy, outgoing, and energetic, the faint stripe up the middle of her chest the only clue to an extraordinary metamorphosis within. When we felt she was mature enough to discuss it, we asked permission to carry out a magnetic resonance imaging (MRI) scan to show us how the remodeled heart had developed. What we found was quite extraordinary. Apart from the double orifice mitral valve, the heart appeared normal, as did the new left coronary artery. Only a thin scar showed the position of the line of stitches up the heart. Remarkably, all other scar tissue had disappeared. The whole inner lining of the left ventricle had been pure white scar tissue. Now all gone. This provided some of the first evidence that an infant's own cardiac stem cells can regenerate heart muscle and actually remove fibrous tissue. Adult hearts cannot recover in this way. What if we could identify and culture stem cells that could do the same for an adult heart? Could this provide a solution for the hundreds of thousands of adult chronic heart-failure patients with coronary artery disease? Like my grandfather. We could inject the cells at the same time as their coronary bypass surgery. Or through a catheter within the heart. But what cells would we use? Where would we find them? How could we preserve and transplant them? One day I would find out.

Now age eighteen, Kirsty is a vivacious and athletic teenager. Had she died, we would never have known about this potential for heart regeneration. Her case could potentially save countless other lives.

nine Domino Heart

> I will give you a new heart and put a new spirit in you;
> I will remove from you your heart of stone and give you a heart of flesh.
>
> —Ezekiel 36:26

H ARDLY A DAY GOES BY WITHOUT A VISIT TO THE PEDIATRIC ICU—to see the babies or small children I had operated upon; to reassure the parents that one day things would get better. More often than not, these visits provided a window on another personal tragedy. Nothing could be worse than the black gangrenous limbs of infants with meningitis. Needing hands or legs amputated. Or children injured on the roads with multiple injuries or brain death. Or complications of cancer and chemotherapy. Or hydrocephalus— babies with huge skulls full of fluid, heads heavier than their bodies, unable to lift them from the bed. Fragile, miserable lives.

It was three weeks after our success with Julie. This time I was summoned by the pediatric cardiologists who wanted to discuss an urgent case. Would I come right away? Several doctors were stand- ing at the foot of the bed, sifting through charts and test results. The desolate mother sat hunched by her son, her face strained with the anxiety of it all, holding a sweaty hand and staring at the heart monitor. The boy was propped up on pillows at 45°. Eyes closed, chest heaving. Making grunting sounds with every breath and coughing intermittently. I could see that he was pale and limp. His eyes were closed, with head tipped back, neck extended, struggling to breathe. Somewhere else in his mind. Quite obviously emaciated with that yellow tinge of terminal cancer. So why did they need me? Maybe he had a tumor in his heart. Rare, but I had operated on several heart tumors in children. Maybe cancer had spread from kidney or bone to the pericardium, causing fluid to compress his heart. I was often asked to make a hole in the pericardium for such cases. Whatever the problem, it looked desperate.

I went unnoticed for a while. Unusual for a cardiac surgeon. I just stood behind them and listened. His name was Stefan. He was ten but looked younger. Mother described him as "not right" for some time. He couldn't keep up with his friends and wasn't concentrating at school. Had stopped playing soccer. If he ran a few yards, he was gasping for breath. Over the school holidays, his parents had become increasingly concerned. Now he was extremely unwell. When the GP listened to his chest, he said it sounded "wet." They sent him straight up to the hospital for an X-ray. The news was bad. The lungs were wet because his heart was huge. He had left ventricular failure and fluid on the lungs. What we call pulmonary edema. It all came out of the blue. There was no previous medical history. No congenital heart disease. Nothing to explain why he was now dying. The whole atmosphere was so tense, I needed to cut it somehow. I said, "Good morning. Can I help with anything?" It was met by the usual response from Archer. "Ah, Westaby, what kept you? Can I show you an echo?"

Stefan was concentration-camp thin, with no fat on his chest wall. It told me that he had been sick for months. Mom wasn't thin, so this wasn't deprivation. But thin provides good echo pictures.

The problem was immediately clear. Both ventricles were dilated, worse on the left. The huge left ventricle barely moved, and the mitral valve leaked. The two mitral leaflets were pulled apart, as what should have been a conical heart turned into a sphere. A rugby ball heart much like Kirsty's. My thoughts were galloping ahead. They were going to ask me to repair the valve and take the back pressure off the boy's lungs. But any attempt at conventional cardiac surgery would finish him off. I didn't say this. I kept my lips closed so as not to alarm the parents. Then I realized where this conversation was heading. It was about pumps. By now, everyone knew about Julie. She was still in the hospital but recovering well. We were beginning to get calls for help from all over the country. Viral myocarditis with chronic heart failure was Stefan's likely diagnosis. Because he had been sick for months, not days, if I performed the procedure, he was unlikely to recover as Julie had. My immediate response was that he needed a new heart. Soon. At the time only the Great Ormond Street Hospital was doing children's transplants. I knew the surgeons well. I used to work there. So let's get Stefan into their system. Onto the urgent waiting list. Simple.

But not so simple. They had already talked to the London transplant doctors. Sorry, but they were pressed for beds and already had several urgent patients waiting. And no, there was no chance at all of a transplant by order. Not in a child. Of course they would get back to us when the situation improved. But in the meantime, "do your best." Stefan was already receiving high doses of intravenous drugs to make his heart pump harder. And diuretics to draw the water off his lungs. Without adequate blood pressure, the kidneys won't work. They were already struggling. He was on the verge of falling off the edge. Into the abyss. Then came the direct question. Could I use another AB-180? With Julie, we had set the precedent. If it was myocarditis, we might save him. And save his own heart. Or at least keep the boy going until Great Ormond Street could take him. It was the family's last hope.

I was conscious that the poor mother was listening to every word. The nurse had a hand on her shoulder—trying in vain to keep her calm. All eyes were on me. I went quiet and thought for a moment. Yes, we did have a second AB-180, but no, it wouldn't work. That inflow cannula was too big and too stiff to fit into a child's left atrium. I shared this response with the disappointed group of physicians. Long, serious faces while mother started to cry. Archer had already suggested to her that the pump was the only outstanding option. If the situation deteriorated further, as it was bound to, his course would be rapidly downhill. Into the grave. I had effectively delivered the death sentence.

Stefan was an ordinary kid from a working-class family. He should have been in the school playground with his pals. Not propped upright and petrified in an intensive-care bed. He was feeling exhausted just lying there. The effort of breathing left him worn out. Then that tedious cough with the tight feeling in his throat. Like being strangled. He felt cold, yet the sheets were damp with perspiration. Strangers were sticking sharp needles into his arms and neck. Sucking out his blood. Shoving rubber pipes up his private parts. Things he should never have had to contemplate at that age. Seeing his mom and dad upset clearly disturbed him. He heard words that he didn't understand. Eventually, things began to drift away into the distance. He was light-headed. Reality was fading. Morphine took the dread away.

Mom and dad slumped on either side of the bed. Leaning forward to be closer to him. Tense and emotionally drained. They should have been at work, not in the hospital. They would rather have been anywhere else but here, without control or influence as their only son lay dying. How could this happen out of the blue? What did they do wrong? They had been told the brutal facts, that the odds were poor. The word *transplant* and Great Ormond Street had been mentioned. But nothing happens quickly. They could see he was in shock and his other organs were failing. Time was their enemy.

Fear gripped their throats. It lay heavily on the chest. Heart-rending, gut-wrenching misery. Sentences become difficult. Then words. Impossible to speak without an outpouring of emotion. Try not to cry in front of the child. Leave that for the end.

Dr. Archer was stressed. Frustrated. He knew the Great Ormond Street doctors well. But also understood that miracles are hard to come by. Other children were waiting in the same situation, with their own desperate parents. Soon it would be too late. He sifted through the blood tests. The potassium was rising. And so was the lactic acid. He would neutralize it with sodium bicarbonate. But Stefan would soon need kidney filtration. Archer did everything to prevent a catastrophic change in heart rhythm. That would certainly precipitate death. What else could he do in this hopeless situation?

The intensive-care consultant waited in the background. He had seen it all before. He looked after many children who died. He could only do his best. Soon Stefan would need the ventilator. He was gasping for air. The morphine further depressed his breathing. So the consultant was hovering with anesthetic drugs and breathing tube. At the same time, he was waiting to do the ward round. He had nine other sick babies and children to worry about.

And then there was Stefan's nurse. Pediatric intensive-care nurses are a special breed. Not everyone can face heart-rending anxiety and distress at work every day. A mature lady with children of her own, she liked to look after my heart surgery babies because they got better. She didn't like to watch children die. Clearly, she felt for these parents. The strain was beginning to show. Someone needed to do something drastic or it would be too late. Her young patient's life was ebbing away. She was the one who pressed Archer to find me.

The atmosphere around the bed was as thick as fog. That sense of impending doom. No one can snatch a donor heart out of thin air, especially for a child. Only a handful of children's heart transplants were done each year. So they looked to me for an alternative. But it wasn't going to happen. I stared at the grieving parents and felt horribly useless. How would I feel in their position? If one of my own kids were in the shit like this, struck down without warning? Undoubtedly having children of my own sensitized me to the plight of anxious families. By then, my daughter, Gemma, was twenty, and I had a son, Mark, at school in Oxford. Same age as Stefan.

Some would suggest that empathy is the key to being a good doctor. The key to compassionate care, whatever that means. But if we really considered the enormity and sadness of every tragedy played out in this unit, we would all drown. My intensive-care colleague needed to get on with his ward round. Not get sucked into the tragedy of Stefan's demise.

By now I was rattled. I really did not want to watch this boy die without making an effort. At the time there was just one ventricular assist device suitable for children. It was called the Berlin Heart and had been introduced only recently, fortunately by my great friend Professor Roland Hetzer at the Deutches Hertzzentrum in Berlin. This was the benefit of scientific meetings. I would call him and ask for a big favor. Maybe tell him that Stefan was German. It sounded that way. And Roland was an Anglophile. Luckily, he was in his office, so I got through at the first attempt. "Roland, I need a Berlin Heart. The boy is ten but small for his age. There is a chance that the heart might recover, but he won't last much longer. What will it cost me?" I knew that the money would have to come out of my charitable funds. The response was as expected: "Let's worry about that later, when do you need it?" Brief pause. "Could you get it to me by tomorrow morning, with one of your guys to help?" Roland was pleased to agree.

The Lear jet landed at Oxford's airport at 8:00 a.m. In the interim, I had sent a message to our new hospital chief executive with a copy to the medical director to announce my intentions. The previous chief executive, the insightful Nigel Crisp, who had backed my circulatory support endeavors, had moved to London by then, and it was only three weeks since I had been threatened with being fired for saving Julie. Archer bravely went to see them both to try to persuade them it was Stefan's only option. The collective body of opinion agreed that the boy could be dead by the end of the day. He had tried the conventional channels. They couldn't help. If Westaby had a solution, they were morally obliged to let me get on with it. Action first. Recriminations later. By the way, had they visited Julie Mills on the ward? A world's first for Oxford. If not, why not? Archer was and remains a religious man. He held back from the "resurrection from the dead" analogy. Westaby was not God. He might even be an irritating son of a bitch. But his job was to save lives, and that is what he was trying to do. So back off for now. Let the Germans come.

Personally, I held fast to the concept that it was ethical to save lives whatever it takes. I didn't need an uptight ethics committee to cast doubt on that. And I didn't care about getting fired. I needed to work where I could fulfill my potential. If Oxford couldn't hack it, I would go somewhere else!

The Berlin Heart consists of an orange-sized blood receptacle, divided by a flexible plastic membrane into two parts, blood on one side, air on the other. Forced inflation of the air chamber moves the membrane and pushes blood onward through the valved tubing. Simple but effective. The pumping chamber sits outside of the body and can be exchanged if blood clots are detected within it. Inflow and outflow tubes connect a pump to each side of the heart, and all tubes pass out through the abdominal wall—from the failing heart to external pumps. Then both ventricles are bypassed and rested with guaranteed blood flow to the lungs and body. Just what the doctor ordered, I guess. Now I needed to get Stefan down into the operating theater. Not only that. The Lear jet was waiting to take the German team home after the surgery. And I was paying for it. Not exactly a taxicab with the meter running.

Stefan had managed to survive the night without being put on the ventilator. Now he was physically exhausted and scared. Even at ten years old, he had an appreciation of his predicament. He could read the concerned faces and his mother's tears. So there was an emotional separation in the anesthetic room. As I said, I prefer to avoid that added pressure. I took the German team to change into operating theater gear. That was embarrassing in itself. We had a scruffy room jammed full of gray lockers; brown wooden benches with paint peeling off; plaster coming adrift from the walls of the toilets. Discarded, blood-scattered theater shoes, masks, and clothing everywhere. What shoes would they wear? We searched around until we matched a couple of pairs. Then went to the perfusionist's room to show them the kit. Desiree was already there. Ready to learn. The surgical residents were waiting with Katsumata. There was an air of frenetic excitement, an appreciation of breaking new ground. Something to tell their partners and kids about when they went home. Would it be on the news tonight? No. Would I be fired? Quite probably. That would make the news. But we would say nothing at this stage. Let's just get the boy better.

Stefan was a sorry sight as he was wheeled in on the operating table. So thin. Pathetic even. At that point I was sure that it wasn't viral myocarditis. This could only be severe chronic heart failure, heart muscle pathology that was unlikely to recover. Step one was still the same. First keep him alive, then take stock. I ran the saw up his sternum and cranked the edges apart with the retractor. We opened the pericardium and tagged the edges to the skin, bringing the heart up toward us. Straw-colored fluid spilled out. I reckoned that about one-fourth of his body weight was excess heart-failure fluid—edema. Full of protein and salt now discarded by the mechanical sucker. I wondered if I was also a sucker to get involved in this world of misery. There were easier jobs.

Now I had a good view of the struggling, dilated organ. A tense blue right atrium. Ready to burst through high pressure in the veins. Making his liver big. The right ventricle was distended. I looked carefully for the left coronary artery, to rule out the possibility of Kirsty's problem. But it wasn't. Archer would have spotted that if it had been. And there was no scar in the huge left ventricle. Just pale fibrous-looking muscle that had given up. Not swollen and acutely inflamed like Julie's heart. I would biopsy the muscle. Then we would see precisely what the problem was under the microscope.

The Germans were looking over the drapes at the top of the operating table. As two of Roland's elite transplant team, they had seen many similar struggling hearts in Berlin. They used the generic term "idiopathic dilated cardiomyopathy." Unusual at Stefan's age. It was already clear that he would need both right- and left-sided support to keep him going. A left heart pump alone would deliver more blood to the body, but it all comes back through the veins to the right ventricle. The right ventricle wouldn't cope. It would pack up. He needed right-sided support. So there would be four tubes coming out through the abdominal wall to two air-driven prosthetic ventricles that passively fill, then forcefully eject blood. Providing similar volume and pumping rate to a normal child's heart. Good, or what?

I sensed his weakened organ would not tolerate manipulation. We would provoke rhythm changes. Make things worse before the pumps could be connected. So I would put him on cardiopulmonary bypass first to keep him safe. I tried to lighten the atmosphere with a joke. "I just deleted all the Germans from my phone. Pause. Now it's Hans free!" They didn't get it. Neither did Katsumata. We pressed on in silence. Made the four stab holes to bring the cannulas out of the chest. Then fixed one end to the relevant parts of the heart and the other to the pump. And most important, we emptied the system of air. I tried another joke. "What's the difference between a hippo and a Zippo? One is very heavy. The other a little lighter!" Again not a titter.

All was completed according to plan. Time for the switch-on. The prosthetic pumps were like normal ventricles but outside the body where you could watch them work. Lub-dub, lub-dub, lub-dub. Energetic and effective. Stefan's own heart emptied. Like a deflated balloon. There was much better blood pressure now with vigorous pulsation in the aorta and pulmonary artery. Lub-dub, lub-dub, lub-dub. An outstanding result. A ridiculously simple approach, but a triumph of life over death. There was something more aesthetic and satisfying about pulsatile flow, but in this case the pumps had to be external. At least continuous flow devices were small enough to implant within the body.

Katsumata took care to ensure that there was no bleeding. He squirted biological glue around the incisions, which stopped the tedious oozing. We needed to leave two drains in Stefan's chest to let the blood out, so now there were six tubes sticking out of his fragile little body. Multiple stab wounds, but all necessary. The usual thick stainless-steel wire stitches were used to draw the edges of the sternum together. Pulled tight and twisted. To cover all the hardware inside. Then back to the pediatric ICU. The first ventricular assist device they had ever encountered. It could have been intimidating for the nursing staff, but it wasn't. We told them, "Don't focus on the tubes or the knobs on the console. There is no need to change anything. Just take care of the boy." He would be alarmed and agitated when he woke up. Make sure that he doesn't pull on the tubes. His lifelines. Best to sit him up and take him off the ventilator. Get the tracheal tube out. One less cause for discomfort. Then it would be possible to reason with him. Easier to keep him calm. His parents could sit with him, and Desiree would be there to help. Close by, even when she was off duty.

With that, the Germans were gone. We were on our own with the new technology. No problem. Stefan improved rapidly. As anticipated, he woke up in the early evening and had the tracheal tube taken out. He was pretty pissed off. Even with his poor mother. But he was pink again with rosy cheeks. His legs were warm. And the hands his parents held so tightly. He was not happy about the "aliens" emerging from his belly. Pulsating away in front of his nose. Priceless lifesaving technology, but daunting for a kid.

As the days passed, I was eager to know what the biopsy showed, so we could work out the next step. The Berlin Heart would keep him alive for weeks or months. But could his own heart recover? I suspected it wouldn't, so in the background we needed to plan for a transplant. Ever curious, I went to the pathology laboratory myself and asked to look at the processed specimens from Julie and Stefan— the same way I always went to the autopsies of my patients who died. The pathologists knew me well enough. And they appreciated clinical feedback. Julie's heart muscle was densely infiltrated with the white blood cells that respond to a viral infection. Called lymphocytes. Viruses are too small to be visible under a light microscope, but the lymphocyte infiltration tells you that they are there. Millions of them, so the muscle was swollen and edematous with the inflammatory process. Not so with Stefan. Much of his muscle was replaced with fibrous tissue. Scar, but not from lack of blood supply. No white blood cells. This confirmed chronic idiopathic dilated cardiomyopathy. Nothing would improve with rest. He had simply reached the end of the line. Julie and Stefan only had one thing in common. We got there just in time. The way forward was now clear. Stefan needed someone else's heart to go home with.

In those days, as now, neither an individual hospital nor a surgeon could organize a heart transplant. Not even if a suitably matched brain-dead donor was lying in the bed next to Stefan. The UK Transplant Service had decided that in order to make better use of scarce donor organs, with equitable distribution, the "urgent" category of patient should be abandoned. So, at the time, donor organs were offered to the transplant centers on a strict rotational basis. Many of those who received a donor heart were still out in the community— not on a life-support device like Stefan. We now know that these ambulatory patients gain little or no survival benefit from a transplant, and many died from complications afterward. Those were wasted organs and one reason I was driven to find an alternative. What's more, if a heart transplant took place involving an organ offered informally, then the transplant unit concerned had to report it to the Transplant Service. That unit would then be placed at the bottom of the waiting list.

I grew increasingly concerned about finding a heart for Stefan. I had to get him into the Great Ormond Street system. I called the transplant surgeon Marc de Leval. I had trained with him and respected him greatly. He was supportive of the fact that I developed a congenital heart service from nothing at Oxford. Equally, I would send him any complex case where I felt he could do a better job. There is no place for pride or arrogance when operating on small people. I explained that we had already tried to transfer Stefan before he took a dive. Marc already knew that, so he was willing to help. He was also interested to see a Berlin Heart. While stable, Stefan was in a parlous and unpredictable state. He could be added to the Great Ormond Street transplant list just as if we had managed to transfer him a week before. But there was a problem. Transfer to London on the Berlin Heart would prove unreasonably hazardous. The ambulance service could not guarantee sufficient electrical power to cover the transfer time. We could not risk getting caught in traffic or having a mechanical breakdown. So we would make the preparations with the Oxford transplant coordinator. Confirm the blood group. Arrange the tissue typing. Look for unusual antibodies in his blood. If we found a suitable donor heart, we would transplant him in Oxford. Now the medical director would have a stroke.

The "end game" came sooner than we expected. But we were ready for it. Stefan had improved day by day. He was still feeble physically but no longer in heart failure. That next weekend, we received the transplant alert. Only thirty miles down the highway, Harefield Hospital was preparing for a heart-lung transplant in a teenager with cystic fibrosis. The cystic fibrosis patient was severely debilitated and dying from lung failure. She had been on home oxygen for several years but was now bedridden, blue and gasping for air. She had high pressure in the lung circulation and regularly coughed up blood.

When she received a heart-lung transplant, her own strong heart could be given to Stefan. This was the plan. A donation of this kind was known as a "Domino Heart."

The cystic fibrosis patient was brought into Harefield while the organ retrieval team stood by. Complex logistics. The heart-lung donor was many miles away, and four separate surgical teams would be involved. For heart and lungs, liver, and two kidneys. All heading for different cities. Vultures hovering above the prey. Ready to consume the body, albeit with the best intentions. All traveling in the night and not without danger. Airborne transplant teams had been lost before in bad weather.

The process would begin Saturday night when it was clear that the heart was a tissue match for Stefan. The two patients had the same blood group. Could anything be better than that? We could operate in Oxford on a quiet Sunday morning. With minimal fuss. Better still, the heart was not subject to the adverse physiological consequences of donor brain death. Head injury donors had often been subject to fluid restriction and diuretic therapy to reduce pressure in the skull. This, together with pituitary gland damage, often prompted the need for continuous resuscitation with several liters of fluid. Many such donors needed massive drug support to maintain adequate blood pressure. As a result, their compromised hearts often failed in the transplant recipient. I had worked at Harefield Hospital for three years and knew the score.

The Great Ormond Street transplant coordinator would keep us abreast of the timing. The "Domino Heart" would be removed from the heart-lung recipient at around 7:00 a.m. and by the time the donor heart arrived in its plastic bags and cool box, Stefan's chest would be reopened and ready. Prepared to go onto the heart-lung machine to remove the Berlin Heart. Ready to cut out Stefan's useless organ, cannulas and all. My team was in early and raring to go.

Ten was a difficult age to face an event like this. Stefan understood the situation, expressing both relief and resignation. And trepidation.

He hated having four tubes the size of hose pipes sticking out of his belly. And the noisy pulsating discs in front of his nose. Blood streaming up one set, then down the other. Bright red in one side, blue in the other. But he was thankful. We had persuaded him that he might need months with the equipment. So the early transplant was a happy release. We didn't tell him the risk of not getting through, which was 15 to 20 percent in those days. From failure of the donor heart, infection, or rejection. But this donor heart was particularly strong—from a live person with a normal brain. Domino transplants were rare then, nonexistent now. And it was a reasonable match on the tissue typing. No alarm bells. We just needed to get on with it. Stefan's parents had been sitting with him since 6:00 a.m., and awake most of the night. Getting progressively more worried but hopeful at the same time. As the tension mounted, they were transmitting anxiety to the boy.

I took Marc to meet the parents. By now they were with Stefan in the anesthetic room. There wasn't a lot of space with all the equipment. Marc's eyes kept diverting to the Berlin Heart. At this stage, it was the only ventricular support system suitable for small children. Great Ormond Street needed to get one so that lives were not wasted. Katsumata came to the door with news. The donor heart had left Harefield. With Sunday morning traffic, it would arrive in Oxford in thirty minutes. Time for Stefan to be put to sleep. The moment of parting had come, which was acutely distressing for the parents and briefly for the boy. Kate, the anesthetist, was poised and ready. Anesthetic was injected into the drip and his pain was gone. A nod from anesthetic nurse Louise and the parents shuffled out the door, huddled together. Their anguish would continue for a while. As if there hadn't been enough already.

After that, things happened quickly. The clock was ticking. After prep, we unpicked Stefan's skin stitches, cut through the sternal wires, and carefully inserted the retractor amid the many pipes. As with all sternal reentries, there was blood clot and fibrin adherent to the heart and tubes. We peeled it off and sucked it away, then washed the heart and pericardium with warm saline solution. Everything needs to be clean. A tidy house for the new occupant. Then we had to find space for the cardiopulmonary bypass tubing. Once attached, we could switch off the Berlin Heart, cut through the tubes close to the heart, and remove them from the surgical field. But we were not about to do that without the donor heart in the room. There could still be a disaster en route. A road-traffic accident. Or someone might drop the heart on the theater floor. It had happened before in Cape Town with Christiaan Barnard. His brother Marius dropped it between the donor in one operating theater and the recipient next door. Oops!

At 9:15 a.m., the heart arrived in its box surrounded by bags of ice. We set it down on its own table. Unpacked it carefully, one bag after another, finally allowing it to rest in a stainless-steel dish. It sat there in salt solution at 39.2°F. Cold and floppy. Like a sheep heart on the butcher's block. But we knew how to revive it, had confidence that it would start again and do its job. So I told Brian to switch off the Berlin Heart and go on to cardiopulmonary bypass. Stefan's own heart emptied out for the last time. It flopped down useless in the back of the pericardium. Marc started to trim the donor heart while I chopped through the four plastic cannulas. Katsumata pulled them out of Stefan's body and threw them away. It was time to cut out Stefan's own sad heart and make ready for the new one. Out it came. The empty pericardium was a curious sight. No heart. It must have been scary when Barnard did it for the first time. Like a car without an engine under the hood.

The donor heart was implanted in a strict sequence. It was essential to align it correctly without distortion. This may sound obvious, but any donor heart is slippery and wet. Not easy to hold in position.

It helps to have a clear three-dimensional vision of the finished product. I am lucky in that respect. I inherited co-dominant cerebral hemispheres. This means that I can operate with either hand. I am a right-handed writer but a left-handed batsman. I preferentially kick a ball with my left foot. Co-dominance helps with many things, but especially surgery. It's more important than the ability to study and pass exams. But a heart transplant is quite simple. Take deep, full, thick bites of the thin atrial tissue and keep stitching. Carefully, so there can be no leaks. The clock is ticking. With the heart sewn in place, the clamp on the aorta can then be removed. This marks the end of the "ischemic" period, the time during which the heart doesn't have coronary blood flow after removal from the donor. Which is a critical time that affects survival. We know that the heart transplants that do best come from young donors with a short ischemic time and blood group compatibility. But that doesn't help much. The patients have to take what they can get, being lucky to receive a heart at all. That is why even "marginal" donors are accepted these days. The over sixties, the smokers, even those with some types of cancer. But it all looked good for Stefan. Blood coursing through the coronary arteries brought the heart muscle back to life. It turned from flaccid and pale brown to almost purple, stiffened and fibrillating. As it began the recovery process, we made the last join between the severed pulmonary arteries. Then more efforts to remove air.

We rested Stefan's magnificent new heart for an hour on the pump. It defibrillated spontaneously and started to eject blood. Gathering strength with time. It separated with no problem from the bypass machine, a precious organ that might easily have gone into the medical waste bin with the diseased lungs. The wonder of modern medicine.

Now we had two important risks. First was the rejection of the donor heart, should the immunosuppression prove inadequate. At the same time, excessive immunosuppression provides the risk of serious, even lethal, infection. So when Stefan recovered, he needed to go to the experts at the transplant center at Great Ormond Street. We had done our bit by keeping him alive. Marc would let us know as soon as a bed became available. Archer and the pediatric ICU helped us to take care of Stefan for the next week, during which he made a remarkable recovery. Then he was transferred to London. We kept in touch and followed his progress. He had a few transient rejection episodes that soon got better with more drugs. Then a virtually uncomplicated recovery from a difficult start. We are still following him almost twenty years later. Now he has his own little family. He has reaped the benefits of an ideal donor heart transplanted quickly, thanks to my friends in Berlin and Great Ormond Street.

Those few balmy weeks in summer—they were epic pioneering days. We had achieved the United Kingdom's first bridge to recovery in viral myocarditis with Julie. Then the world's first pediatric partial left ventriculectomy in Kirsty. And now the first bridge to transplant in a child. These were dire emergencies undertaken on the hoof. Worked through in the dead of night with my dedicated team of overseas fellows. Great Ormond Street adopted the Berlin Heart for their heart transplant program, initially with charitable funds. Too much to expect the NHS to pay. Then it became the only approved system to support babies and children with severe heart failure in the United States. It still is. Needless to say, we never got to use it again at Oxford. Children with heart failure either reached Great Ormond Street in time or they died. Julie and Stefan emptied out my research funds. But what price can you place on two young lives?

ten   Life on a Battery

> We will now discuss in a little more detail the struggle for existence.
>
> —Charles Darwin

IT WAS A WARM SUMMER'S MORNING IN THE FIRST WEEK OF June at the turn of the millennium. At 11:00 a.m., there was a tentative, almost apologetic, knock on the door. There stood Peter, his large frame filling the doorway. He leaned on a stick, swaying and sweating profusely. Head bowed, panting for breath. Out of pride, he refused to be pushed through the office door in a wheelchair. Only weeks before, he had received the last rites. But details still mattered to this man. Desperately trying to disguise his distress, he slowly lifted his head and stared straight ahead through the doorway. His lips and nose were blue. He couldn't see me yet, but he reminded me of a concentration-camp victim. Hope gone long before. My secretary, Dee, was visibly shaken by Peter's distress. I broke the silence. "You must be Peter. Please come in and sit down." Hidden behind the stooped frame was Peter's foster son, who parked the wheelchair in the corridor. I tried to lighten the mood. "Did you pay for that parking space? This is the NHS, you know!" They didn't get it.

Peter shuffled slowly through to my room, then began staring at my certificates, awards, and other professional paraphernalia on the walls. He was checking me out. A religious man, he had worked as a counselor for the terminally ill with AIDS. Now he faced death himself. His existence had become that of an intelligent mind attached to a body rendered useless by heart failure. He was expecting the end to come soon. The sooner the better. I gestured to the armchair. He set the stick aside and sat down with a grunt. Now I was checking him out. He was breathless on the slightest exertion. His belly bulged with engorged liver and fluid. I could see that his legs were swollen and purple. He wore oversized sandals with socks stretched over massively swollen feet. There were stained dressings on leg ulcers that the socks failed to cover. I didn't need to examine him. This was gross end-stage heart failure. I was amazed that he had made the effort to leave home. He could die at any moment.

Some months previous to Peter's visit, Philip Poole-Wilson and I had written an open letter to members of the British Cardiac Society to announce that we were ready to implant a revolutionary new type of artificial heart. The Jarvik 2000, which we'd tested extensively in the laboratory. We needed to recruit terminally ill heart-failure patients who were ineligible for cardiac transplantation. At fifty-eight, Peter Houghton fit the bill.

I had already read his medical notes sent from his cardiologist. Peter had been first diagnosed in March 1995 with idiopathic dilated cardiomyopathy. It had been triggered by a viral illness that affected the heart muscle. Another bout of influenza that turned to myocarditis. He had initially recovered. Or so it seemed. Now he had an enlarged, flabby heart, an irregular heart rhythm, and a leaking mitral valve. Such patients usually die within two years of diagnosis. Peter was well beyond this. He had been admitted to the hospital on many occasions, gasping for breath and coughing up fluid. Without rapid treatment with diuretic drugs, this "water on the lungs" would be his terminal event.

On each occasion the drug treatment had been escalated with modest and short-lived relief. Now he had reached maximal levels of all useful drugs and his single kidney was failing. Months earlier, his cardiologist had asked the surgeons at a London hospital whether they would repair the leaking mitral valve. This raised Peter's hopes until the outpatient visit. Then the surgeon was dismissive out of hand. "No way. It's far too late for that. Too high risk." Now, he was unable to lie flat and could only sleep propped up on pillows or sitting in an armchair. Exactly as I remembered my poor grandfather.

In my office, Peter was still sweating. He tried to regain enough breath to speak. I remember thinking, *This man would be lucky to survive a haircut. Are they really expecting me to operate on him?* But that is what mechanical hearts are for. This was precisely the intolerable existence that they were meant to improve, the lives they aimed to prolong. By now Dee had composed herself and had brought tea. Peter thanked her. Now we could talk.

I thanked Peter and his son for making the huge effort to come. Then I asked him the circumstances of his referral. He had been working as a psychologist at London's Middlesex Hospital. Ironically, he was writing a book called "Healthy Dying." Just days before, he had struggled to a meeting with his coauthor Dr. Robert George. Rob was a palliative medicine consultant at University College Hospital. Peter wanted to say a last good-bye but was in so much discomfort that Rob went to find a cardiologist to see if anything could be done. While waiting for his colleague to finish with a patient, Rob read the cardiologists' notice board and saw a cutting about the heart-pump project at Oxford. He recognized the name of the surgeon, Steve Westaby. He had known me as a junior doctor. They wondered whether I could help Peter.

Coming directly to the point, I suggested that we could help each other. To be blunt, I needed a guinea pig. I had the opportunity to do something that had never been done before—something that had the potential to help patients worldwide if it worked.

I took the Jarvik 2000 out of a desk drawer to show them. This titanium turbine was the size of my thumb, or a C battery. I explained that the pump would fit inside his own failing heart, implanted at what used to be the pointed apex. His left ventricle was now so large that there was plenty of room. We would sew a restraining cuff onto the muscle, and that would hold the pump in place. Then punch a hole through the heart wall and slide the pump in. The high-speed turbine would empty his struggling heart through a Dacron graft and into the aorta, the major blood vessel to the body. I showed him how the torpedo-shaped impeller spins within the tube. Unbelievably fast. It pumps as much as a normal heart but with continuous flow. And no pulse. The only potential problem: The right side of Peter's heart would have to cope with the boosted circulation. If the right ventricle held up, this manmade pump could be as good as a transplant. If it didn't, Peter would die.

Peter winced at the word *transplant*. No one should underestimate the profound psychological trauma of being turned down for a transplant, the patient's last hope when life approaches its end. He was bitter. He had been through the selection process twice. The first time he was told that he wasn't sick enough for a heart transplant. The next time, age fifty-eight, he was told he was too sick.

I tried to put this into context for him. Assessment for a heart transplant is a brutal process. To describe transplantation as the "gold standard" treatment for heart failure is equivalent to claiming that a lottery win is the best way to make money. To begin with, heart transplantation is ageist. In the 1990s, patients older than sixty years were not considered. There were around 12,000 severe heart-failure patients younger than sixty years of age in the United Kingdom but fewer than 150 transplants. It was the transplant physician's responsibility to select patients who would accrue most benefit. And there were precious few of them.

What I wanted to do was to help patients in Peter's position—the desperately ill who would never get the transplant opportunity. Those of all ages who were abandoned to "palliative care," to the use of narcotic drugs to blunt the misery of an unpleasant and lingering death. Peter had refused that option. He told me that he was well familiar with death. He had comforted more than one hundred patients in the last days of their life. "Telling them the things they need to do, can do, the stages it will take, things like that," he explained. It wasn't the time to share body counts. By then, I had already dispatched more than three times that number to the afterlife.

Now rested, he had the measure of me and was more animated. An extraordinary character began to shine through the morbid preamble. His smile penetrated through the gray veneer of disease and the purple nose. I warmed to the man. So traumatized was he by repeated rejection that he had no expectations from our meeting. On the contrary. He expected to be turned away.

I had serious doubts that he could survive an anesthetic, but if we took him on, no one could claim that we had picked an easy patient, one who didn't *need* the pump. Both my own hospital's Ethics Committee and the Medical Devices Agency had requested independent verification that the first patient be terminally ill and with very short life expectancy. No one would argue that Peter didn't meet those criteria. So the decision rested with me. Impulsively, I told him that it would be a great privilege if he would allow us to help him. That if he wanted the first pump, it was his. There followed a look of astonishment that evolved into a broad grin. This was his lottery win.

He asked about the odds. I said around 50–50 but knew that to be optimistic. Like many patients, his main worry was that he would be left brain damaged and worse off. I reassured him that if the operation didn't succeed, he would definitely die. Strange way to reassure someone, but he was taken by the concept that failure spelled death. Life was unbearable. But like most Catholics in his position, he wouldn't contemplate suicide for his family's sake. Surgery was an option for euthanasia without the moral debate. I asked about his wife. Why had she not come with him? Diane was a teacher and couldn't get away on short notice. Together they had founded the National Association for the Childless and written *Coping with Childlessness*. They had looked after thirteen foster children. As a younger man, he had played rugby. Something we had in common. I felt that he was a good person, and one to make the best of his extra life.

I showed him the equipment and asked whether he could cope with life on a battery. He would have to carry the controller and batteries at all times. They would fit into a shoulder bag. There was an alarm that sounded when the batteries were low or disconnected. They would need changing twice each day. He would literally plug himself into the main electrical source at home overnight, every night. Very futuristic.

Now the next surprise. Dr. Jarvik and I had worked out a revolutionary new method to bring electrical power into the body. The big issue with the electrical power lines of other pumps that emerged through the abdominal wall was their propensity for infection. Constant movement of the cable through fat and skin allowed bacteria to enter. Sometimes even the pump became infected. Seventy percent of patients who lived long enough were eventually troubled by this. And many needed further surgery. Instead, we planned to screw a titanium plug into Peter's skull. The scalp skin is virtually free from fat and has a generous blood supply. Because the plug would be rigidly fixed into bone, there would be no movement to disrupt the skin's healing around the titanium pedestal into which the external power cable is inserted. We believed that this innovative approach would minimize the risk of power-line infection in the long term.

So Peter would have an electric plug in his head, carrying electricity to the pump through a cable in the neck and chest. I would be the real Dr. Frankenstein. Not some movie freak.

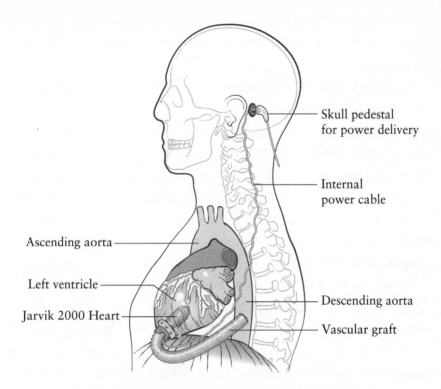

The Jarvik Heart Pump with Skull Pedestal

Peter laughed. His mood was changing. I explained that he would have a large, painful incision around the side of the left chest to implant the pump. Not so funny. There would be other small incisions in the neck and scalp to fix the electrical system. Peter asked whether this had ever been done before. I said no. He would be the first to receive a "lifetime" implant. We would be the pioneers.

"So, would it work?" he asked me.

"Yes. I've done it in sheep."

He laughed again and asked whether he would hear or feel the pump in his heart.

"The sheep never complained."

It occurred to me that I should warn him that he would not have a pulse. Like Julie with the AB-180, the blood would be pushed

continuously through his body. Life would be different, but arguably preferable to the inevitable alternative. He was a guinea pig in
this respect.

He asked another intuitive question. If he lost consciousness
away from the hospital, how would anyone know whether he was
alive or dead? This was moving away from my comfort zone. I side-
stepped a speculative response. But he was right to ask. Months later,
in winter, another pump patient fell and hit his head at home. He
was found some time later unconscious, cold and pulseless. The ambulance crew thought he was dead and took him directly to the mortuary. I never knew whether they were correct. Did they turn the
pump off and feel for a pulse again? I doubt it.

Now Peter's last question. Was I nervous about attempting the
operation? A procedure that was pure science fiction, quite likely
to snuff him out. My response. "Absolutely not. Not if you want
me to do it. I'm not the nervous type. Doesn't suit the job." These
words prompted a direct response. "Let's go for it then." I told him
that he should take some time to discuss it with his family and
friends.

There was one more thing. I needed to see echo pictures of Peter's heart myself. We pushed him around to the Cardiology Department and helped him up onto the couch. Breathless again. We could
soon see why. His huge left ventricle was massively distended. Barely
moving. The mitral valve was held open by the stretched heart wall,
but this wouldn't matter with the pump in. The pump simply sucks
blood through—as long as the aortic valve doesn't leak, and it wasn't.
To me, the right ventricle seemed to be working well enough. All in
all the anatomy looked good for the surgery. I just needed to stop
focusing on the risks. Failure was not an option. Death in the first
patient would destroy the program.

Peter got himself down from the couch and insisted on walking
to the door. It would be wrong to imply that he had a spring in his
step. But he left with something more important. Hope. Hope for

the first time since staggering away from the transplant assessment in despair. Now we simply had to get on with it.

Peter's wife, Diane, and some of the foster children took part in emotional discussions. Should Peter hang on for the short time he had left or risk dying in surgery for the chance of a better life? Diane told her husband, "I can't make the decision for you or tell you what to do, but whatever you decide I will support it." Two days after our meeting, Peter confirmed that he would consent to the operation. Now I needed to ask Philip Poole-Wilson, Europe's leading heart-failure cardiologist, to confirm Peter's poor prognosis. He could come to Oxford late on the evening of June 19. We would proceed with surgery the next day.

I had to coordinate the team from Houston and New York. Bud Frazier, who had undertaken the animal work at the Texas Heart Institute, would be an important member of the surgical team. He had implanted far more mechanical hearts than any other surgeon. Dr. Jarvik would bring the device from New York. We would admit Peter to the hospital two days before the operation. We needed to optimize his heart-failure treatment and teach him how to manage the controller and batteries. It was equally important that other members of the team should get to know him.

On the afternoon before surgery, we brought Peter to the cardiac ICU. Desiree Robson, our chief nurse, shaved the left side of his head in preparation for the skull-pedestal incision. Dave Pigott, the anesthetist, inserted a cannula into the artery at the wrist. Then a large-bore venous cannula into the internal jugular vein on the right side of Peter's neck. He then floated a balloon catheter through the veins across the right side of the heart and into the pulmonary artery.

I brought Jarvik and Frazier to visit Peter in the early evening. The conversation was animated and uplifting for a man who faced 50–50 odds in less than twelve hours. For the first time in months, he talked about his future. What he could do to support our program if he survived. And where he would go for his first holiday in

years. Positive stuff that helped all of us. Now we needed the professor to arrive.

Philip arrived from Heathrow Airport at 10:30 p.m. He talked
at length with Peter, looked through the data, then emerged just
after midnight. He wished us luck. Adrian Banning, Peter's cardiologist at Oxford, likened his predicament to that of a man on a diving
board who was about to jump but had no certainty that there was
water in the pool. Later, he reflected, "Houghton was functionally
dead. All he had left was a mind full of frustration. Heart failure has
a worse prognosis than any type of cancer. Once you have fallen off
the threshold for the transplant waiting list, conventional medicine
has little to offer. Every cardiologist has clinics full of these people,
unable to work, just hanging on, waiting to die."

We all met in the anesthetic room of Theater 5 at 7:30 a.m.
As usual, Bud arrived in Stetson and cowboy boots. I asked Peter
whether he had any reservations or last thoughts. He replied that
he would be in a better place after the surgery. One way or another.
I glibly told him that he would be fine. That's what every patient
should hear before being anesthetized.

Once Peter was asleep, we positioned him left side up on the
operating table with the side of his head and neck exposed. I marked
the anticipated site of the surgical incisions with indelible black
marker pen. We would bring the power cable out of the apex of the
chest, through the neck and to the left side of the head. My cochlear-
implant-specialist colleague, Andrew Freeland, would screw the
titanium plug to the skull. Meanwhile, we would expose the pericardium and aorta through the left chest. This needed a large incision
between the ribs.

With a degree of trepidation, I exposed the leg artery and vein
in the groin to attach the heart-lung machine. Then I performed the
chest incision through fat and wasted muscle. The metal retractor
cranked open the ribs, bringing the lung and pericardium into view.
Behind the lung was the aorta. Through a separate wound on the

shoulder, we passed the black insulated power cable up into the neck. Then through the neck and out behind the left ear. Difficult, as there was some important clockwork in proximity—large arteries and veins, not to mention the vital nerves.

On the end of the electric cable was a miniature three-pin connector. Literally. This was inserted through the titanium plug that had six screw holes to fix it rigidly to the outer table of the skull. Andrew made a C-shaped incision behind the ear and scraped the fibrous surface off the bone. Then a power drill was used to make the screw holes in the skull. We worked meticulously but were making it all up as we went along. The plug was screwed securely onto the skull with dry bone dust incorporated to promote healing around the titanium. All that remained was to punch a hole through the center of the skin flap through which the percutaneous pedestal part would protrude. We could then attach the external power line leading to the batteries and controller. That done, we closed the head and neck incisions, now ready to implant the pump itself.

I opened the sac around the heart. It was a sorry sight. The huge quivering left ventricle was more fibrous tissue than muscle. It barely moved, and by now, an hour into the surgery, Peter's blood pressure was uncomfortably low. Lactic acid was building up in his blood. We had to start the bypass machine to support the circulation. Bud held the thumb-sized titanium pump while I pulled the lung forward to expose the aorta. We needed to sew the Dacron vascular graft, which emerged from the pump, end-to-side onto the descending aorta in the back of the chest. Then the pump itself could be implanted into the heart. And the graft had to be just the right length. Not so long that it could kink. Worse still, too short. What's more, the stitching had to be pristine to avoid bleeding. Once done, we were ready for the big event. We started to stitch the restraining cuff onto the rounded apex of the heart, which resembled a rotten melon. Never again would Peter's heart bear sole responsibility for his circulation. From now on, his life was reliant upon technology.

All that was left now was to cut out the plug of heart muscle through the center of the cuff, and then slide in the pump. Like coring an apple and sliding in a flashlight battery. This was Peter's life raft. We were about to create a pulseless human being. So far it was going well. I cut a cross in the muscle encircled by the cuff, and with a coring tool, we punched out the hole and slid in the pump. It was in. The plan worked. So far.

Desiree was holding the controller and batteries, waiting for the instruction to switch it on. When I was satisfied that there was no more air in the pump or vascular graft, we turned up the pump speed to 10,000 rpm. A flow probe showed that it pumped 4.5 liters per minute. We then cut back on heart-lung machine flow to let the combination of the device and Peter's own right ventricle take over. As we slowly shifted support from one system to the other, I finally told Brian to "come off." The whole process had taken two hours.

Peter's huge left ventricle was sucked empty and the aortic valve remained closed. We were all fixated on the monitor screen. The arterial pressure trace was an absolutely flat line, measuring no more than two-thirds of normal blood pressure. Pressure in the veins was also less than normal. Although this suggested that the right ventricle was managing well, it was too low. It was important to have the circulation well filled, otherwise the powerful turbine could suck the left ventricle empty and obstruct. We aimed for a balance whereby the pump did most of the work but Peter's left ventricle continued to eject some blood.

We needed to adapt our treatment strategy to a new, pulseless physiology. Flat-line physiology. We had looked after a lot of sheep, so we knew just how to handle it.

The remaining and most troublesome issue was to stop the bleeding. Every cut surface and every needle hole was oozing blood. Peter's distended liver had not been making clotting factors, an issue common to most patients who needed artificial hearts. So we fed in donor clotting factors and the sticky cells called platelets that plug needle holes, and we left the residents in charge of closing Peter's chest. That alone took several hours before the bleeding abated.

Having removed gown and gloves, we reviewed the power consumption: 7 watts, and pump flow that oscillated between 3.5 and 5.5 liters per minute. The rate depended upon the pump rotor speed and Peter's own blood pressure, which was providing resistance to pump flow. This was counterintuitive physiology: when Peter's blood pressure increased, flow decreased substantially. But right now things were okay. The pump was doing its job.

With the chest closed, the drapes were taken off and Peter was moved onto the trolley for transfer to the ICU. We had an elite nursing team, carefully prepared and versed in what to expect. Peter was hooked up to the monitor. An audience gathered to see the flat-line patient, the first to be fitted with a revolutionary new type of artificial heart on a permanent basis. We left the nursing team in charge, with orders to call us if anything went awry. Then away to the hotel bar with my American colleagues.

I was overstimulated after one of the most exhilarating operations I'd ever performed and could barely sleep. So when the sun rose at 4:30 a.m., I visited Peter in his room. Listening to his heart with a stethoscope, there was no lub-dub, lub-dub, just the characteristic continuous whirr of the pump rotor. His single functioning kidney had stopped producing urine, but we expected that. What worried me most was that blood transfusion is bad for the lungs, and he had already had 30 units of the stuff. With blood now sucked out of his own left ventricle and flowing backward up the descending aorta to the brain, I wondered how long it would take him to wake up. Only time would tell.

Peter remained stable for the next thirty-six hours and began to regain consciousness. As soon as he was sufficiently awake to breathe, cough, and understand instructions, we propped up his large frame and took out the breathing tube. The first thing he said when he saw me was, "You bastard." A thoracotomy between the ribs is very painful and he had other incisions in the head, neck, and groin. But it was said with a smile on his face. He was glad to be alive. We talked for a while. About how the operation had gone. I joked that despite his Christian faith he was now Frankenstein's monster. Powered by the bolt in his head. The thing that was currently giving him the headache. He was motivated to get well and make the most of his new life.

Within the first week, his kidney function had improved and we no longer needed to give him dialysis. He worked hard to get out of bed and mobilize with the physiotherapists. Whereas the pump immediately restores blood flow to normal levels, it still takes months to reverse the debilitating wasting effects of chronic heart failure. It is the same with a transplant. But already it was a source of wonder and relief that the breathlessness had gone. There was no more back pressure from the failing left heart on his lungs. He began to lose liters of fluid that were chronically accumulated in his tissues. The leg ulcers began to heal. His face and nose were pink, not blue.

Remarkably, Peter left the hospital on the eleventh postoperative day. Taken home to Birmingham by his family. That was record speed, something that could never happen in the United States, where ventricular assist device patients spent many weeks under surveillance. There was a press conference with many photographers waiting at the hospital entrance. Peter enjoyed this. He was in his element. Our Anglo-American team had achieved a world's first, but Peter was the star. The bionic, pulseless man. He described himself as the model "cyborg."

Peter's ability to exercise increased progressively. Within weeks, his belly began to shrink as the fluid around his guts dissipated. Then his huge legs became slim again. At an outpatient appointment five months after the operation in November, even his heart rhythm was back to normal.

He was newly chatty, saying that "events since June had taken him from the position of a refugee, forced to pack up and abandon the trappings of his existence, to that of a man given uncertain leave to remain." His engaging personality shone through. He had shifted from inexorable fear and bewilderment to undisguised pleasure at avoiding death.

Peter was fitter and healthier than he had been in years. "It really annoys me when people say I was brave; I wasn't brave at all," he said. "I was swapping a certain slow death for the risk of a quick one, or the chance of a complete recovery. When I first left hospital I didn't dare plan ahead. I was literally living my life from one day to the next. Now I am thinking about what to do with my time, and contacting all my friends to tell them I'm not dead."

Out and about in Birmingham, Peter was a curiosity. It took time for the hair to grow back on the side of his head. At first the plug and external black power cable were obvious to passers-by. Children would come to him to ask why he had a bolt in his head. Was he a robot? So happy was Peter with his new life that he was willing to stop and explain things to them. He had a particularly happy Christmas that he never expected to see.

During the January sales, he was out shopping when he felt a sharp and painful jerk at his head. A would-be thief had snatched what he thought was a camera bag but it contained Peter's controller and batteries. The skull-pedestal connector was avulsed and disconnected. The pump stopped. The teenage mugger attempted to flee with bag in hand, but the power failure alarm sounded noisily. Sensing a trap, the young thief discarded the bag and ran off. Shoppers helped to retrieve Peter's power cable, and he fumbled to get the power line reattached to his head as fast as possible. An old lady sorted it out for him but was bewildered by what she had achieved. Reconnected, the pump whirred undeterred. Peter recalled, "I did feel faint but I think it was more the shock than anything else. The wrench to my head really hurt for several days."

Aside from that one frightening episode, Peter regained a relatively drama-free existence. He spent the first year getting as physically well as possible. Then spent the second finding some meaningful purpose to make his "extra life" worthwhile. This second chance would constitute more than 10 percent of his overall life span. It was vital for him to have a goal for his existence beyond being an exhibit. So he worked tirelessly to raise money and draw attention to our efforts. He was desperately eager for others to benefit from the same opportunity. Soon Peter became an integral part of our team, counseling other potential assist-device patients and their families.

Peter was never the most compliant of patients. He suffered from nosebleeds and would unilaterally reduce his anticoagulant dose to cope. There was a price to pay for his reprieve: he needed to change batteries every eight hours, recharge them, and carry the equipment everywhere as a matter of routine. Sometimes Peter would forget to change the battery before going out, and on one occasion he was in the middle of a dental filling when the battery near-expiry alarm went off. The dentist had to drive him home.

He was a prolific writer. He published his own book, entitled *Death, Dying, and Not Dying*. He gained considerable satisfaction when his charity was able to contribute to pump implants for other patients. Then greatly enjoyed the camaraderie that emerged from his new bionic colleagues. Most of these patients resumed active and sometimes adventurous lives. Skiing, sailing, surfing, and sex.

In the background, he always hoped for sufficient native heart recovery to allow removal of the hardware. Although this happened to a point, we resisted the temptation. This was fortunate, as his heart eventually deteriorated again and for the last three years of his life, he was wholly reliant on the device. Ironically, he was offered a cardiac transplant in his home city but pointedly refused to discuss it.

In his sixth and seventh extra years, he was troubled by aging problems that he never expected to encounter. He developed rheumatoid arthritis in the hands, which hindered his writing, and his prostate enlarged to the point that it required surgery. We arranged this for him in Oxford, because no other hospital would operate on a patient in his circumstances. As Peter put it, "I wonder if one day the burdens of living a worthwhile life might come to outweigh the wonder of it."

On his last trip to the United States in August 2007, Peter gave an interview to the *Washington Post*. He admitted that his artificial heart brought about some religious crises. It caused him to think about his Catholicism. Questioning the very afterlife, he wrote, "Who knows? These are only priests. They are not very good at being challenged on the subject." He went through bouts of clinical depression. "Several times I thought it would be better if I wasn't here. Let everyone else get on with their lives. I felt I'd like to put an end to it. But choosing the method put me off. I felt cowardly about killing myself." He talked to a psychiatrist about suicidal thoughts. "He advised me to try and think about what I was doing without being prohibitive. He challenged me—are you sure you mean it? I did mean it, but not sufficiently to overcome my fear of the actual process." Peter was prescribed anti-depressants for eighteen months, but he never took them.

My endearing cyborg was drifting in no-man's land. Seven and a half years after the implant, we were way into uncharted territory. Previously, no one had survived with a mechanical heart for more than four years. As Peter put it, "The procedure lands you in a position that no-one has ever endured—what life on a battery does to you as a person. You're an invented entity trying to cope with it, trying to deal with the emotional context of it. You become cold hearted." He admitted a careless attitude toward money. "You don't care if you have overspent on your credit cards or not. If you don't have any time left you might as well enjoy it. You think, what the hell, if I want something I'll have it."

Much of the money Peter raised charitably he spent on visits to international conferences. Everywhere he was a revered figure. A driving force behind the new technology. Yet the last paragraph in the *Washington Post* piece was revealing: "Things get normalized. You no longer see yourself as odd or outside the norm. Being snatched from the brink of death and transformed into a poster child for cyborg life, despite serious psychological transformations, has been quite an experience. A roller coaster. Better than being dead I think. Three days out of five."

By now, Peter had a job with the Birmingham Settlement to help the homeless and poverty-stricken. At the same time, he was working to establish a spiritual retreat in the mountains of Wales. He had undertaken a ninety-one-mile charity walk, hiked the Swiss Alps and even the American West.

However, within weeks of the *Washington Post* article, Peter died. I was away in Japan, working to introduce ventricular assist devices in a culture that did not accept transplantation. Peter's death was not pump or heart-failure related. He simply suffered a profuse nosebleed that stopped spontaneously but caused his single diseased kidney to fail. He could easily have been put on dialysis, which we had previously done with him for a week after his first operation. But the local hospital declined to intervene. Without treatment, the levels of potassium and acid in his blood caused his own heart to fibrillate, and the pump was switched off. Had I been in the country, we would have taken over his care and treated him. I regarded it as a wholly unnecessary death.

We asked Peter's wife, Diane, for permission to perform an autopsy to elucidate the long-term effects of pulseless circulation. The pump itself was pristine. There was no blood clot and minimal wear on the rotor bearings. We returned it to Rob Jarvik in New York. It continued to work for years on a bench-testing apparatus. Peter's own left ventricle remained hugely dilated—still functionally useless. The only finding related to the pump was the thinning of the muscle layer in the wall of the aorta. As Peter had little or no pulse pressure, his aorta did not need the thickness of muscle that the rest of us have. A perfect example of how nature adapts to its circumstances.

Peter left an important legacy. The experience confirmed the enormous potential to provide a good quality of life for the many thousands of patients with severe heart failure who are not eligible for a transplant. There are few if any ethical dilemmas, however hard you search for them. The patients targeted for this treatment would otherwise have short, wretched lives.

Our "dead man walking" lived for almost eight years after his operation. As a result, the United States and many European countries adopted these miniaturized rotary blood pumps as an alternative to cardiac transplantation. Many patients went back to work and contributed to the economy. Yet there was no chance that NHS patients would benefit. Saving money took priority over saving lives. The UK transplant units saw their exclusivity threatened and talked the technology down. Self-interests before the patients' interests. An unfortunate surgical trait. Sixteen years later, with accumulated expertise in managing pump patients, we are on course to achieve equivalent survival between mechanical hearts and heart transplantation. I was pleased to play my part in that.

Peter made it clear that extra life is not ordinary life. There is a price to pay and a second dying to come. But he was the first to reveal the true potential of blood-pump technology. It was something that most believed to be impossible. He was a truly remarkable man.

eleven Anna's Story

Body and mind, like man and wife, do not always agree to die together.

—Charles C. Colton

.

M Y WORK IS TO HELP OTHERS AT THE MOST VULNERABLE stage of their lives. When they meet me, they all know that they could die. Some expect to. One lady was so certain of it that she made it happen after a straightforward operation. Never underestimate the human mind. It is a powerful force.

One thing is for certain. For the patient and family, every single professional contact is emotionally charged. None more so than for Anna. Anna had a difficult start in life. Her mother died when she was only eleven months old. She was fortunate to have two other strong characters in her life. Her father, David, brought her up in a peaceful Oxfordshire village, close to the church—not just geographically. Later, her husband, Des, was a huge source of support through her troubles.

Seven months after Anna was born, her mother suffered an extensive stroke—completely out of the blue, in her mid-thirties. Why this happened at such a young age was never explained. It was the last contact she had with her baby daughter. When David was told that his wife was dying, he went straight home to wash the diapers.

Yet Anna recalls a happy childhood. Holidays in Yorkshire or Guernsey. Sunday afternoon walks. Picnics and outings. David taught her about nature and the great outdoors, and she found an affinity for birds and plants. She worked hard at school but found religious and social activities in the village much more appealing than books. Above all, she adored small children and babysitting. In church, she was the one who held the new babies, the one who rang the bells—a long-standing family tradition.

Like my own mother, Anna left school and became a bank clerk. She started early in the morning and often worked late. She put her heart and soul into everything. As her father put it, "Anna's inner strength and perseverance likely came from my influence and I am proud to accept it is so."

Anna met her husband, Des, when he was walking his dog in the village. They fell in love, got married in July 1994, and bought a house. She was twenty-five and happy both at home in the village and at the bank.

Soon after their wedding, Anna started to feel tired, at times absolutely worn out. She put it down to long hours at work. Then there were inexplicable bouts of sudden, severe breathlessness, which she attributed to panic attacks. For no discernible reason, a sore red spot appeared on her toe. It blistered and became infected. Antibiotics fixed that, but what could have caused it? Unbeknownst to Anna at the time, these were the classic symptoms of a rare and life-threatening condition. The same one her mother had suffered from. But no one took the trouble to find out. Life took over.

At 9:00 a.m. on August 29, Anna was in bed nursing a violent headache. Not a hangover—she didn't drink. Des was reading the newspaper downstairs. She recalls that *Skippy the Bush Kangaroo* was on the television. The room started spinning, and she was losing touch with reality. Going to a strange and different place in her head. She just managed to shout out to Des downstairs. Asked him to call the doctor before everything went black. Anna could hear Des on the telephone. The anxiety in his voice worried her. She felt she needed an ambulance. Her brain knew what she wanted to say, but her voice and mouth wouldn't respond. It was as if her brain had been transplanted into a different, lifeless body. It was terrifying.

Anna was rushed directly to the John Radcliffe Hospital in Oxford and appeared to be both unconscious and paralyzed on arrival. The paramedics wheeled her straight into the resuscitation area. "Airway, Breathing, Circulation" is the rescue algorithm. The medical ABC. Every doctor, nurse, and paramedic learns this.

The doctors passed a tube into her windpipe to prevent her from choking to death. Then started to breathe for her with the mechanical ventilator. Her pulse was steady and strong. The blood pressure elevated. High blood pressure that goes with brain injury. So the circulation part was fine. Or was it? Did anyone listen to her heart? Did anyone notice the blistered toe? Was her mother's death factored into the equation? There had been no time to look into the family history yet. It was a matter of saving Anna's life first, then establishing the cause of the catastrophe.

Diagnosis is like a jigsaw puzzle. You need to find the pieces first, then fit them together. Only then does the full picture emerge. Anna had suffered a sudden catastrophic brain injury. In young people, this is usually caused by a bleed into the brain from a congenitally weakened and ruptured blood vessel. But there is a potential second option—an event known as paradoxical embolism. An embolus is a piece of foreign material floating around in the bloodstream. Paradoxical embolism occurs when a blood clot breaks off from the veins in the legs or pelvis but instead of floating to the lungs, it passes through a hole in the heart and continues upward to reach the brain. This can cause a sudden and sometimes fatal stroke. Anna needed a brain scan with a view to emergency brain surgery. There was one positive sign, however. Her pupils were normal size and reacted to light. She was not brain dead.

The brain scan was performed with injected dye to show the arteries within the brain. Magnificent architecture, like the branches of an oak tree. Here was a tree of life with one branch sawn off, one critical vessel that came to a premature full stop. There was no bleeding. It was an embolus, lodged in a critical artery supplying the brain stem. Flow to that important nerve center was curtailed.

A crucial mass of white matter was already dead. It included the nerves to the arms and legs, the nerves controlling speech, together with nerves governing the body's automatic reflexes. All damaged. She appeared to be deeply unconscious, and probably blind.

Why could Anna hear and think, when she appeared to be gone? Like being buried alive in a coffin with a window. The dreaded "locked in" syndrome. Complete paralysis of voluntary muscles in all parts of the body except those that control eye movements. Only vertical movements of the eyes and blinking remain. Yet there is no damage to the thinking brain—the cerebral cortex—the gray matter. Such patients remain alert and fully conscious. They can think but are mute and immobile—a nightmare scenario.

Anna never did lose consciousness. Her vocal cords were not paralyzed, but the ability to coordinate breathing with speaking was lost. To the outside world she was in a deep coma, but from Anna's perspective, her hearing and thought processes carried on normally. Understandably, this trapped new life was terrifying. She could see out, but there were always complete strangers around her and she could hear a persistent intermittent beep—the monitor. As her nervous system lost control, she felt cold inside even though she was covered in warm blankets. It was as if her body had been frozen and strapped down.

She recalled an olive-skinned man in a green top and trousers who was trying to put a cannula into a vein in the back of her hand. He seemed to be digging around, and it hurt. She couldn't move a muscle or make a sound, but she was screaming inside. He didn't speak to her. It was as if they were in two separate worlds. Anna wondered if she might be dead but being experimented on. Where was God or Heaven now?

Meanwhile, the doctors tried to figure out where the embolus had come from. If it originated from leg veins, there had to be a hole in the heart—to let it through from the right side of the heart to the left. Many normal people have a small hole left over from the fetal circulation in the womb between their right and left atrium. It's there to divert blood from the right heart to the left before the lungs expand at birth. Anna needed an echocardiogram, the ultrasound examination of her heart chambers. All stroke patients should have one. Not least so further similar episodes can be prevented by closure of the communication.

Anna's scan told the story. It linked her own fate with her mother's early demise. There was a huge tumor filling her left atrium. It was fragile-looking, like seaweed, but forced into the mitral valve every time the atria contracted, effectively obstructing the left side of her heart. This explained her breathlessness and fatigue.

The infected toe also began as an embolus, a small piece of the fragile tumor that broke off as it pounded into the valve, then was flushed to her toe. The next fragment went north, not south. Directly through the carotid artery to the basilar artery and the brain stem. A catastrophic route. A self-destruct sat-nav couldn't have done it better.

I had operated on many heart tumors, rare though they tend to be. Anna had a myxoma, a common but benign type that are often fragile like Anna's, so bits break off. Many cause stroke as the first symptom. For this reason, they are operated upon urgently. And most myxomas never come back after removal.

The cardiologist, Dr. Forfar, wanted me to remove it as a matter of urgency. I was moved by the story and the sight of her lying paralyzed in the bed. Her eyes were open, with a blank stare. No movement. No response. Ironically, when I held a stethoscope to her chest, I could hear the murmur of an obstructed mitral valve and the "plop" of the myxoma into the orifice. Had no one listened to her heart before? At that stage, we didn't know about her neurological prognosis. We tend not to operate on patients after a recent stroke. The anticoagulation for the heart-lung machine can cause more bleeding into the brain. On the other hand, there was the likely risk that more fragments of tumor would embolize soon and prove fatal.

It was a decision for Des and David, Anna's husband and father. Did they want me to do it even if the prognosis was poor? An impossible choice. They were shell-shocked. David had lost his wife, and now his precious daughter was in the same situation. They both wanted Anna to have a chance. What did I think? I felt there was nothing to lose by operating. When they decided on the operation, I took her to the theater that same afternoon.

Anna had a small, vigorous heart. Beating away, looking entirely normal from the outside. On the inside, it was a land mine primed and ready to explode. It was important not to touch it and disturb the delicate fronds of tumor before their escape route could be blocked by a clamp across the aorta.

First, we went onto cardiopulmonary bypass to support the circulation and empty the heart. Next, I applied that clamp to stop blood flow to the coronary arteries. Cardioplegia solution stopped it altogether. Heart surgery is simple—or should be. With the little heart lying flaccid and cold, I opened the right atrium.

The myxoma was attached to the other side of the partition between the right and left atria known as the atrial septum. The safest way to approach it was to cut away that septum and locate the base of the myxoma. Often there is a short stalk between the septum itself and the mass floating in the blood. The aim is to remove the whole thing so it can't grow back. Which is best done in two steps. Cut the stalk and lift the fragile lesion out gently. Without breaking bits off.

Then excise the whole base. That is precisely what we did. I proudly dropped the tumor into a container of formaldehyde preservative. A present for the pathologist to check that there was no malignancy. I had operated on patients whose benign myxoma grew back and turned malignant. Rare. But it can happen.

With the tumor gone, Anna's heart separated easily from the bypass machine and we closed her up. Now she was safe. Badly wounded but safe from further damage. The surgery itself was not the greatest challenge. As a quadriplegic patient, Anna's ability to get over the surgery was questionable. She couldn't respond to instructions. Would she breathe independently? Could she cough? To lie flat and immobile is a prescription for chest infection or pulmonary embolism from the thrombosis of veins in the legs. We had to work hard to bring Anna through this journey. It was a task for the physiotherapists and her friends and family. They were encouraged to talk to her and play her music, even though there was no sign of awareness. Des put her earphones on to play the local radio station. There was no response at all.

Remarkably, Anna *was* aware of everything around her. As the anesthetic drugs wore off, she could see and hear again, but still she couldn't move. Worst of all, she felt pain that she was unable to communicate. To the outside world, she was still in a deep coma.

One night when Anna was sweating, a new nurse changed the sheets on the bed. In kindness, the nurse stroked Anna's head and said, "I'm sorry I can't do anything more for you." Anna panicked inside, taking this compassionate comment to indicate that she was dying. On another occasion, a less sympathetic nurse said, "She looks dead!"

One day, two nurses were changing the bottom sheet on her bed. As they rolled her from side to side, Anna's recurrently dislocating right kneecap displaced. No one else recognized the fact. Leaving it dislocated was agonizingly painful, but there was no way to let anyone know. Eventually, an observant junior doctor spotted the strange asymmetry of the knee and put the patella back in place. No anesthetic. Nothing.

Des and father David visited every evening after work, hoping to see signs of improvement. I passed by her intensive-care bed several times each day. It lay on the route between my office and the operating theater. My immediate thought was that she had severe and irrecoverable brain injury. But I'm no brain doctor.

Nine o'clock in the evening, Monday, September 5. Anna's uncle was visiting and trying to talk to her. The tape that kept the eyelids down to prevent the surface of her eyes from drying out had been removed. Suddenly, Anna opened her eyes for the first time. Her uncle jumped up in surprise, shouting, "She's awake, she's awake, Anna's awake!" Not only that. She could follow the movement of a finger up and down with her eyes. This was the first indication of consciousness since the stroke a week before.

Des and David had just left the hospital, having been there most of the day. When they heard the news, they rushed back but by then Anna had fallen asleep. With the realization that Anna was not brain dead, it was reasonable to let her try to breathe for herself. In the next twenty-four hours, we managed to remove the breathing tube from Anna's throat. A great relief for her. It also made physiotherapy and bed changes easier.

A few days later, Anna was awake for most of the day, breathing well, with stable pulse and blood pressure. There was the usual pressure to free up intensive-care beds, and against the family's wishes and my own grave reservations, she was transferred to a single room on the ward. With less frequent chest physiotherapy, she soon developed pneumonia, which needed treatment with a combination of antibiotics. Still prostrate and unable to cough, this was a life-threatening situation. A high swinging temperature, profuse sweating to the point of dehydration, and uncontrollable bouts of shivering made Anna's life intolerable.

The pneumonia was getting worse. Then, by chance, Des saw the letters DNR scrawled across the brown folder of her medical notes. Do Not Resuscitate. This had been written without any reference to the family, on the grounds that her projected quality of life would be unacceptably poor. It sent the family a clear message that the medical staff had given up.

Specifically, they would not put her back on the ventilator if the chest infection proved overwhelming. David said about this, "I think it was put on her records when she was moved out of the ICU. I am not certain of the ethics but felt they should have discussed it with us." Of course they bloody well should have. Vets don't let pets die without discussing the issues with their owners. It might have been reasonable to mention it to her family.

Now Anna was in a single room on the ward, and she was solely my responsibility. Not the intensive-care doctors. I called a case conference with my own surgical assistants, the ward nurses, and the physiotherapists. Then I brought in Des and David for a frank and open discussion. We had come so far with Anna. She was awake, and though the prospects of neurological improvement were limited, the family wanted her to have the best chance.

What did "Do Not Resuscitate" actually mean? With the myxoma gone, she had a normal young heart that was never going to stop. No one was going to have to pound on her chest or zap her with the defibrillator. What she needed was physiotherapy and antibiotics for a while. And loving care to make her feel human again. The pep talk served its purpose. The team pulled together and cured the pneumonia.

Gradually, she remained fully alert for longer periods and was able to sit in a chair. Her breathing improved, and she learned to communicate by blinking, could make yes or no responses to questions. Well-meaning nurses worked out a system for others to communicate with her through winks and blinks. But unhelpfully, they taped the instruction sheet onto a locker too far away for Anna to see it. No one thought to put her glasses on. Eventually, she regained some ability to control her head movements. Then learned to use a specially devised "speech board" to interact with visitors. The process was slow but gave her a means of expressing her well-preserved intellect. In time, she began to tell us her own story.

I remember waking up in what I assume was the middle of the night. It was very dark. There was that intermittent beep all the time and what looked like lots of televisions lit up. I now know they were the heart monitors in Intensive Care. It felt like my neck was resting in a bowl. Someone was pouring lovely warm water over my hair and massaging my whole scalp. Whoever it was, they were washing my hair! It felt absolutely wonderful.

When they had finished, the bowl was taken away and I tried to hold my head up. I wanted to see where I was. My neck seemed to have lost all its strength and the back of my head felt as if it had been filled with concrete. I couldn't speak and don't remember being able to cry at all. I was frightened. There were curtain rails in a square above me and a painted ceiling. Unable to move or lift my head I just lay flat on my back looking directly upwards. No sign of life in my vision but plenty of voices. One voice I recognized. A woman. My line manager at the bank. I was worried she had come to check up on me. To see why I was not at work. One person mentioned a funeral the next week. I thought it was mine. My uncle realized and reassured me. My brain worked fine. Where was my body?

Often lots of people in white coats gathered around the bed. Always talking about me, not to me. Things I'd never heard of before. Then they just left. I wanted to ask them stuff. Where was I? Why was I here? How dare they talk as if I wasn't there. I was indignant but I couldn't get it across. Much of my confused state and dreadful thoughts could have been prevented if people talked to me. No one explained what had happened to me.

One day a medical resident called Imad came to see Anna from the Rivermead Rehabilitation Center. He was kind and spoke directly to her. He asked if she would like to have the feeding tube through her nose replaced by one inserted directly into the stomach. "I hated the tube in my nose. I opened my eyes wide and smiled to indicate yes. That was the first time I remember anyone trying to involve me in my own care."

Imad was there to assess Anna for a rehabilitation program when she was fit enough to leave the hospital. This was still three months away. She needed to be much stronger and able to swallow before she could leave. Progress was slow but steady. She had a few more chest infections and more courses of antibiotics. At least they removed the Do Not Resuscitate order from the front of her notes. Anna was very much alive and wished to stay that way.

By the end of January, Anna was strong enough to move on. Strong enough to move her head and blink. Although she remained quadriplegic, being able to breathe without a ventilator was a great blessing.

It was almost three years before Anna could move back to her modified home with Des and start rebuilding her life. Easter 1997. She remained physically dependent but mentally alert. On weekdays, Des went off to work early and two helpers would arrive. They got Anna out of bed, after which one stayed with her for the morning. At lunchtime, a different carer came, staying until around 7:00 p.m. Then two others would arrive to help put her to bed. A rigid routine. She got out and about in a sophisticated electric wheelchair directed by movements of her head. To the supermarket and local park. She liked to be treated as a normal person—have people talk to her. From a scripted box of tricks mounted on the wheelchair, she could open and close the front door, draw the curtains, and operate the television. The box was programmed to operate anything with an infrared controller. A nod pushed against a lever on the left side of her head. This triggered a cursor that stepped down a list of commands. When it reached the chosen instruction, Anna nodded on the lever again to select it.

Anna also had a computer room overlooking the garden. In it, a receiver monitored head movements via a white reflective dot fixed to the bridge of her glasses. This enabled her to direct the mouse around the computer screen. With specially created software, she could write e-mails and keep in contact with her friends. Apart from loss of mobility, she professed that little had changed in her personality since the stroke. As a religious woman, she accepted her situation and made the best of it. The local radio station ran a campaign to buy an adapted car that would carry Anna's wheelchair. Her father christened the blue Vauxhall Combo the "Anna-mobile" after the similar popemobile. Her main worry? That she might grow another myxoma in her heart that I couldn't remove. She was content in her own body and didn't want life to be cut short by another stroke.

Dr. Forfar kept her under surveillance every six months with an echocardiogram. The first myxoma had been radically excised and was unlikely to return. But I was aware of genetically based "familial myxomas" and was convinced that Anna's mother had died from one. Patients with the familial myxoma gene can develop further tumors at different sites. I hoped that wouldn't happen.

On August 11, 1998, I had devastating news from Dr. Forfar's clinic. "The myxoma has recurred," he told me. "Anna is very frightened. When can you take it out?" I assured him that if he could bring her into a cardiology bed that afternoon, I would do it tomorrow. It was a re-operation, so we would need to have blood available. Re-operations are always more complex. The sac around the heart is always obliterated by inflammatory adhesions from the first procedure. As I had learned back at the Royal Brompton Hospital, the heart can be stuck to the back of the breastbone. But I had done hundreds of re-operations since that first debacle many years before. It wouldn't be a problem.

Anna was sitting in her wheelchair looking petrified when I saw her on the ward. Des was crestfallen. Dad was on the way. We would meet in the operating theater the following morning. I said everything would be fine, but I needed to go and change my operating list. The emotional black hole was about to pull me in. I needed to escape.

The next day, Des came to the anesthetic room with her. He stayed to keep her calm until she was unconscious. The first time I met Anna she was already paralyzed but still had muscular arms and legs. Now these were markedly wasted by three years of immobility.

I listened with a stethoscope before painting the chest. I was convinced I could hear this one. As suspected, the origin of the myxoma was at a different site. Toward what we call the left atrial appendage. There was no stalk. It had a broad base that I chopped out. Then sewed the atrial wall back together. This time I looked carefully around the rest of the heart to make sure there were no other tumors lurking in the recesses. Nothing. We came off the bypass machine easily, closed up again, and took Anna back to the ICU. We knew she would wake up this time and had her communication mechanisms ready. The physiotherapists were on standby. It was all much easier after the first time. Once again, her family and friends rallied round for her sake. I hoped that would be the last time I saw her.

It wasn't. The third time, Anna was thirty-two and it was seven years since the first operation. On April 10, 2001, her follow-up scan revealed another huge myxoma in the left atrium, this time in a different position, directly above the mitral valve. This tumor was more solid and plopped in and out of the valve orifice. A dangerous situation. Large myxomas can block the valve altogether and cause sudden death. Again Anna and the family were in a state of distress, having watched the echocardiogram unfold on the screen. I took her straight back into the hospital and to the operating theater the following day. With more extensive adhesions, the third time through the sternum is always tricky. One more time, I entered the heart through the right atrium and opened the remains of the septum. The tumor was right there in front of me. Originating next to the mitral valve and partly from the atrial septum. I set about lifting it from the left atrium with an ordinary kitchen spoon. Useful implement for tissue that has the consistency of jelly. I had never seen or heard of a patient needing surgery for more than three heart tumors. Soon we would run out of places on the little heart to insert the bypass cannulas.

Anna bounced, or rather slowly climbed, back again. Her spirit and the support of Des and her dad were extraordinary. She suffered the inevitable chest infection, but the physiotherapists brought her through. We were assiduous about pain control and used the same communication mechanisms as before. This was the benefit of a consistent ward nursing team in those days. She spent three more weeks in the hospital before going home. We learned that she had been struggling with depression. It would be inconceivable if that were not the case. Massive stroke and multiple heart operations. Then the realization that this must have been the cause of her mother's premature death. Worst of all, the persistent anxiety about the tumor recurring. It had happened twice at different sites. Would it happen again? Was a fourth operation technically feasible? Could it be done safely? We all hoped that it wouldn't come to that.

Now Des couldn't bring himself to attend the follow-up appointments. The strain of sitting there watching the echo images on the screen was just too much. Instead he went to the church to pray. Anna was thin. So it was easy to take echo pictures. Clear as day. Each follow-up she lay there desperate to see empty chambers. In atria that were getting smaller with each operation.

On August 5, 2002, sixteen months after the last procedure, there was another nasty surprise. Dr. Forfar called to show me the monster. The largest tumor so far. I didn't believe that a new myxoma could have grown to that size within months. I said nothing but wondered whether this one could be malignant. I had operated on a young woman with that scenario before. The first myxoma was benign. Second time it was a highly malignant myxosarcoma. We didn't want that for Anna. I brought her back into the hospital for an urgent fourth operation.

To obtain written consent for an operation, we are obliged to explain the risks. No one could claim that the risk of death during a fourth-time heart operation could be any less than 20 percent. Equally, there was the significant risk of a further stroke. There was a real chance that bits of myxoma would break off and visit the brain. But if we didn't operate, the tumor would continue to grow rapidly and obstruct the heart. The bigger it was, the more the danger of embolism. It was between the Devil and the deep blue sea. I figured that we were better to take on the Devil. Anna and the family had divine help with that. And she couldn't swim.

On the day of surgery the church held a vigil for her. As always Des brought Anna to the operating theater. I stayed in the coffee room. Des had doubts that she would get through this one.

This was the biggest and most aggressive myxoma so far. Practically filling the whole left atrium. I did a radical excision, then I took a long, hard look at this battle-scarred cavity. Was there anything I could do to stop further growths? I decided to take the electrocautery and kill the cells of the whole inner lining. The layer that was genetically programmed to terminate Anna's life. I fried as much as I could see with smoke rising—like burning the stubble in a cornfield, a scorched-earth policy. I didn't want Anna to succumb to this curse.

As we obliterated the cell lining, I had an extraordinary and unexpected stroke of luck. I pushed open the mitral valve to look around the left ventricle. There was a baby myxoma on one of the muscles of the mitral valve. Too small to be seen even on the best echo. Destined to grow large, had we missed it. Out came the bastard. Into the pot with the rest. Everything to be analyzed by the pathologist.

The heart continued to look good in normal rhythm. Frying the inside of the left atrium had no adverse effects. I watched the rest of the operation over the drapes. With a good team, I wasn't needed to finish off. When the sternum was wired together, I went to call husband Des. Aiming to put the family out of their misery as soon as was reasonable.

There was little bleeding, so the whole procedure was quicker than anticipated. I suspected that Des might still be in the church. I called and told him the battle was over. Again she was safe within the bounds of her ability to bounce back from the trauma of it all. But I was concerned that she might give up if she dwelled on the recurrence issues. Anna needed an overdose of positive thinking, a massive morale boost to get her through the next few weeks. Something to bring her through the pain, the fear, and the uncertainty. So I asked Des to bring God back to the hospital with him. I had seen off the Grim Reaper, for now at least.

Anna recovered slowly. This time without a serious chest infection. Everyone rallied round once more to see her through. All with a gargantuan dose of positive thinking. By now she was a well-known character in the hospital and the community. People were willing her better.

Once again she went home—only to face the inevitable outpatient appointments and the much-dreaded echocardiograms. Months passed without incident. Then years. Two of them, at least. Then came the gray, wet November afternoon the day before Guy Fawkes night. November 4, 2004. The usual appointment at Dr. Forfar's clinic. Anna with her dad. Anna is helped onto the couch for the echo. Adrenaline levels rise in anticipation. Gel goes onto her bony little chest to improve contact with the probe. Within seconds came that familiar sinking feeling. A great view of another lump floating around in the left atrium. Like a goldfish in a jam jar. So much for my scorched-earth policy. This was too much for Anna. Too much for Des and David. It was easy to understand their standpoint. How much could one person endure? Why was God letting this happen? More to the point, where to go from here? How much heart could anyone remove from this young woman? The situation was too emotionally charged to make a quick decision. Anna and her dad went home in abject desolation. The cardiologist had to think about it. He would discuss it with me but let the family settle down for the Christmas period. Of course they couldn't rest. There was no peace of mind. Anna knew this was a death sentence.

They all came back in early February. Des, too, this time. There was no uncertainty for him now. Only the discussion about what could be done, if anything. A repeat echocardiogram was unbelievably miserable. Though all benign, Anna's myxomas grew rapidly. This one was 2 centimeters in diameter. It was already prolapsing dangerously through the mitral valve, so further stroke was likely.

Dr. Forfar called me with the news. What did I think? Would Anna be considered for a heart transplant? Sadly not. A transplant leaves a large cuff of left and right atrium to which the donor atria are sewn. So it wouldn't protect her. A heart-lung transplant could remove the whole heart. But no one would consider that because both lungs were stuck to the chest wall after the previous surgery. I said I was willing to operate again, but we all needed to agree that it would be the last time. Between us, we felt that we couldn't leave Anna to the inevitable.

When asked, the family agreed that she would rather die during the surgery than be abandoned. In the event of success, there would be no more echocardiograms. A head-in-the-sand strategy. No point making everyone miserable again. Anna was admitted on Valentine's Day. Twenty-two years to the day after she and Des were engaged to be married.

This fifth operation was predictably difficult and dangerous. With patience and great care, we reentered the chest and dissected out just enough heart to get back into the right atrium. Having achieved that safely, I went out for a break. This is a good strategy in complex re-operations. A necessary one for surgeons with an aging bladder. Now for round two. I opened the right atrium to approach the left. Intending to go directly through the patch from operation three. At the mouth of the inferior vena cava draining from the abdomen was an unsuspected right atrial myxoma. As large as the one we were chasing on the left. We took it out. It almost fell out. Then we lifted out the left atrial myxoma. Job done again with a great sense of satisfaction. We closed up the heart, removed the air, and warmed the blood. Unperturbed by this fifth insult, the much abused little organ bounded off the bypass machine. Two myxomas for the price of one. Again. We closed the chest over it. Never to be exposed again. Relief for me. Resignation for the family.

At first the postoperative course was straightforward. Anna spent two days on the ventilator, then tube out and frequent physiotherapy. Everyone was elated that she survived. Then she was given some soup without adequate supervision. With the brain stem stroke, her swallowing was always an issue. She inhaled the hot liquid and choked. There followed a long period on the ventilator with a chest infection. This needed several courses of antibiotics and eventually a tracheostomy. But she came through in the end. No worse than before. Anna and Des went home to get a grip on the uncertainty. To try to banish the depression and have the best life possible.

Time passes. We didn't bring her back to the hospital. The rehabilitation center, Rivermead, was hugely supportive and kept an interest in her. Above all, she was well supported by the church and the community. From time to time, I would ask Dr. Forfar whether he had heard anything. As time went on, we both lost track of her. We heard nothing until I discovered that a neighbor knew her well from church. Then I had serial updates. She was happy. Des was happy. He stuck by Anna. Occasionally, I would receive a card.

In 2015, more than ten years after the last operation, the "Anna-mobile" pulled up outside my home. She was in her wheelchair at the back. Beaming and blooming. Des came to the door with a cake. With the carers' help, Anna had made it for me to celebrate their twenty-first wedding anniversary. What happened to the myxomas? The genetic storm had abated. The battle was won. With divine help, I expect. It brought to mind a line from the poet George Herbert. "Who would have thought my shrivel'd heart could have recovered greenness?"

I hope they live happily ever after.

twelve Mr. Clarke

> Before you tell the truth to a patient, be sure you know the truth
> and that the patient wants to hear it.
>
> —Richard Clarke Cabot

Mᴀʀᴄʜ 18, 2008. I ᴡᴀꜱ ᴀᴍʙʟɪɴɢ ʙᴀᴄᴋ ᴛᴏ ᴍʏ ᴏꜰꜰɪᴄᴇ after the first case of the day. A baby with a hole in the heart. Nice result. Happy parents. At the far end of the corridor, a woman stood weeping. She was smartly dressed and had two young children holding on to her coat. This was none of my business. But after forty years in surgery, I am still not immune to other people's suffering. The desperate little tableau upset me. Everyone else strode past them purposefully. Going about their hospital duties. Deadlines, figures, waiting lists. I was about to divert toward my office, and a pile of paperwork. I couldn't do it. Although I looked and felt a mess in my sweaty theater gear, I approached her.

The poor lady was so consumed by grief that she didn't notice. She thought I was a porter waiting for the elevator. Quietly, I asked whether there was anything I could do. After a minute to compose herself, the woman explained that she had left her husband in the cardiac catheterization laboratory. They were told that nothing more could be done. He was dying. Now she needed someone to look after the children. Then she could go back and sit with him so that he didn't die alone.

I pushed her for more information. Her husband, Mr. Clarke, was forty-eight. Earlier that morning, without warning, he had suffered a massive heart attack. First, he was taken by ambulance to the nearest district general hospital, where he suffered a cardiac arrest and was resuscitated and placed on a ventilator. Having established the diagnosis of myocardial infarction, a cardiologist inserted an intra-aortic balloon pump (IABP) and relayed him on to Oxford, more than an hour away, for urgent angioplasty. The objective of angioplasty is to open the blocked coronary artery and stop the oxygen-depleted heart muscle from dying—the infarction bit of myocardial infarction. The cardiologist feeds a balloon catheter through the aorta and into the blocked coronary artery and then inflates it to open up the tiny vessel. Then a small metal stent is inserted to keep it open. In most cases this reinstates blood flow to the compromised heart muscle—a process known as "reperfusion." Now the critical bit: reperfusion within forty minutes of the onset of chest pain salvages 60 percent to 70 percent of the muscle at risk. Beyond three hours, only 10 percent of the injured muscle will survive.

Mr. Clarke had been bounced from pillar to post. This took much more time than was reasonable. The treatment guidelines advise the use of "clot busting" drugs in cases of delay. These can dissolve the blood clot that is blocking the narrowed artery and restore blood flow. Not as good as angioplasty, but better than nothing. Yet all Mr. Clarke had received was a dose of aspirin and oxygen in the ambulance.

Oxford has a fantastic emergency angioplasty service. Round the clock. All day, all night. Once in the cath lab, Mr. Clarke got the best treatment. His blocked artery was opened. But the left ventricle had been badly damaged during the delay, and it wasn't doing any work. There was poor blood flow down the reopened artery and to the rest of his body. A normal heart pumps 5 liters of blood per minute. This heart was managing less than 2 liters per minute. With a low blood pressure of around 70 mm Hg. Half of what was normal. Lactic acid was accumulating in his blood. He had reached the stage we call cardiogenic shock. Sinking fast. Without a miracle, he was doomed.

The poor kids were about to lose their dad. I didn't want that to happen. I said I would see if there was anything I could do to help. Maybe we could try one more thing. Because of our record with circulatory support, I had been sent another new ventricular assist device to test from America. It was time to give it a try!

We agreed that Mrs. Clarke should take the children to the cafeteria. Make an effort to divert their minds from the misery. I would come back to them. I needed to get Mr. Clarke into that operating theater as soon as possible and would have to reschedule the operating plan for the day. We would start by supporting him on the heart-lung machine to improve his life-threatening metabolic state. Then take over from the dying heart.

I started to make my way down to the cath lab past my dismal modular office. My new secretary, Sue, was killing ants on the windowsill. Waiting for me to get to grips with paperwork. Mercifully, there was a new excuse for me to avoid it. I asked that she call the anesthetic room of Theater 5. Warn them about the change in plan. "What plan?" Sue was entitled to ask. She had no idea about Mr. Clarke. Nor was there time to explain. And would she warn the perfusionists that I was going to use the new CentriMag pump?

I wanted to see the coronary angiogram so I knew what we were dealing with. Whether this heart stood a chance of recovery. That only took two minutes. The left anterior descending coronary artery had been blocked at its origin but was now wide open again with a metal stent through it. This prevented it from closing off again.

The coronary flow wasn't as brisk as it should be. The echo showed that a substantial part of the left ventricle was indeed motionless. Not contracting at all, even though the artery was open. The $64,000 question was whether the muscle was already dead—myocardial infarction. Or whether it was suffering from what we call "myocardial stunning." Down but not out. "Stunned" muscle remains alive but takes days or weeks to recover. We would find out if I succeeded in keeping him alive.

There was no chance to explain all this to Mr. Clarke. He was on the way out. He had the ventilator tube down his throat, lying flat on the trolley, and when I tried to introduce myself, it was clear his mind was failing, bordering on unconscious. His kidneys had stopped working. His lungs were filling with fluid. He was icy cold and deathly pale, yet sweating. There was froth in the corner of his mouth, bubbling through blue lips, and his eyes were rolling. This is how heart-attack patients die. How my grandfather had died. There was no time to send for porters to move him. I asked the nurses to head for the elevator. Just get him up there before he arrested. I would deal with the consent form. Whether he lived or died, he would not be suing me.

They say everything in life is about timing. For Mr. Clarke, timing was the stuff of fantasy. You couldn't make it up. My chance encounter with the distressed lady on the corridor. An empty operating theater. And the new pump called CentriMag. Reminiscent of Julie's good fortune with the AB-180. These were the lucky ones. The pump was called "CentriMag" for a reason. The blood-propulsion mechanism—known as the impeller—spins within a magnetic field like a centrifuge. Up to 5,000 revolutions per minute. Mag was for "magnetically levitated." It can pump up to 10 liters of blood per minute without damaging the delicate red blood cells. Far more than needed. This was the challenge for artificial hearts from the outset. Now the technology was improving rapidly.

Mr. Clarke was too sick to linger in the anesthetic room. By now he was a metabolic wreck. He was wheeled directly through to the operating table. To give him a general anesthetic at that point risked immediate cardiac arrest. So the monitoring lines and transfusion cannulas were inserted using local anesthetic. To keep him alive I had to get him onto the heart-lung machine. Then his blood needed filtering to remove acid before we switched to the CentriMag system.

The sternotomy incision was bloodless. Corpses don't bleed. The injured heart quivered, making its final agonal efforts to keep him alive. As always, cardiopulmonary bypass changed everything. The struggling heart emptied. I had a good view of the stiff muscle that had been starved of blood and oxygen. I could see that it wasn't dead. Not black and necrotic. I could even see and feel the coronary stent sitting within the artery. Like a rat in a snake's gullet. Blood coursing through it to the swollen muscle. The ventricle was down but not out.

Mr. Clarke was experiencing a completely standard death from heart attack. It happens to hundreds of patients every day across the NHS. I had a grim determination to show that he could still be saved with the right technology. For the sake of that family.

With the CentriMag system, plastic tubing diverts blood from the left atrium out of the body to an external rotating pump head. A control console the size of an old-fashioned typewriter regulates the pump speed. Then more tubing brings blood back to the chest and into the aorta, where it emerges from the heart. This simple arrangement bypassed the struggling left ventricle and allowed it to rest, at the same time providing generous blood flow to Clarke's brain and body.

By releasing clamps on the plastic, we allowed the tubing to fill with blood. Pushing out air. As always the whole system must be airless. Obsessionally so. Now it was time to switch on the CentriMag. We balanced the reduction of flow in the cardiopulmonary bypass circuit with an increase in the CentriMag system. Then CentriMag took over altogether. A smooth and effortless transition. Like clockwork.

I looked at the clock. It was almost three hours since I had dispatched the grief-stricken family to the cafeteria. They were sitting there wondering whether he was alive or dead. Expecting dead. There was nothing I could do about that now. Good news would make up for it. For once I did the finishing work myself and closed the chest, taking care to protect the life-preserving tubes. By the end, there were two pacemaker wires and four plastic tubes emerging from beneath Mr. Clarke's ribs. Two of these were just drainage tubes to let out blood.

I went to find Mrs. Clarke. By now other family members had arrived and had taken the children away from the hospital. I wanted to bring her to the bedside myself. It was a bit like being in a spaceship. Wall-to-wall technology. The ventilator to breath for him. His circulation supported by the CentriMag. What room remained around the bed was taken up by monitoring equipment and drainage bottles. Amid all this was her husband's broken body. Something to look at, rather than communicate with.

Her first reaction was alarm. An emotional stab wound. I thought her legs would give way. We moved quickly to sit her down by her husband. Her immediate instinct was to hold his hand. Always the same response but at least it was warm now. When she last saw him, it was cold and clammy. This time he even looked pink. Not that grayish-blue color of those dying from cardiogenic shock. The nurses were kind. They scraped Mrs. Clarke from the ceiling and explained the paraphernalia. They were confident enough to manage the equipment. The orders were simple. Don't change anything. We were winning.

After a week, the serial echocardiograms suggested the uninjured muscle looked much better, so I decided to take the optimistic route and take the CentriMag out. So back to the operating theater and reopen the sternotomy incision, wires and all. We slowly reduced pump flow and watched the heart's performance on echo. The left ventricle was ejecting well. Clarke had a normal heart rate and adequate blood pressure. There seemed to be little residual damage from last week's catastrophe. *Bloody brilliant,* I thought. We removed the cannulas and tubing to the pump, washed out the chest, put in clean drains, and closed him up for the last time. He remained perfectly stable. After another twenty-four hours, Mr. Clarke woke up and had the breathing tube taken out. Returned from his week away. Resurrected from the dead. When I finally spoke to him, he recalled nothing of the events. No "out-of-body" experiences or flashbacks. He had no idea who I was. Nor any recollection of which hospital he was in. There was just a line up the middle of his chest that he didn't have before. And the pain.

I wanted to be there when his kids came back. Not with them but away in the corner of the room somewhere. Watching as they came in to see their dad. It was worth the wait. Amazingly, only a week later Mr. Clarke went home. Equally remarkable was the fact that at follow-up three months later, his heart looked normal. All the "stunned" and struggling heart muscle had recovered. A "just-in-time" job.

For me, the Clarke case was a watershed moment. So many patients still died after a heart attack even when emergency angioplasty had succeeded in opening the blocked vessel. We had shown that at last some of these victims could be saved with simple, inexpensive technology. A repetitive theme.

Splint a broken bone and it will heal. Rest an injured heart and it may recover. Not always. But I felt the patients deserved that chance. What's more, the nurses on the ICU found the system easy to manage. Turn up the flow or turn it down. We had control over the patient's whole circulation by turning a knob. More straightforward than driving a car.

Now the sting in the tail. Six months after Mr. Clarke suffered his heart attack, the same thing happened to his younger brother. Age forty-six. I was away at a conference. The second Mr. Clarke was taken to his local hospital, only to be passed on to Oxford. By that time, he was already in cardiogenic shock. The family received the same message: "There is nothing more we can do." They searched out my office, desperate for help. There was none. No surgeon, no pump. The wife lost her husband. His children lost their father. Misery.

Now completely well, the first Mr. Clarke took over their care. When I heard about this, I was desperately sad, yet at the same time I was relieved that I did not have to face that family. With age, my objectivity was fading. Empathy was taking over. I was suffering for my profession.

thirteen

Adrenaline Rush

> We are but tenants. Shortly the Great Landlord
> will give us notice that our lease has expired.
>
> —Joseph Jefferson's headstone

BATTLE OF BRITAIN FIGHTER PILOTS THRIVED ON ADRENA-line, the hormone secreted by the adrenal gland in response to stress. One minute relaxing in the sunshine, the next scrambling for their planes and soaring into the sky. Anticipating the conflict ahead. Risking sudden death. Medical students are taught that adrenaline is the fight-or-flight hormone. Flight as in escape—not flying the Spitfire. There are times when I have to scramble like the fighter pilots. When every minute counts. Even seconds. The call comes that a patient with a penetrating chest injury is on the way to the Accident Department. By helicopter or ambulance. That the entry wound is close to the heart and the blood pressure low. They need a cardiac surgeon as soon as possible. Scramble!

Sometimes simple, frustrating issues spell the difference between life and death. A set of traffic lights, a police car in front, no space in the hospital parking lot. I cannot speed like an ambulance. There is no blue flashing light on my car. I drive fast and get into trouble. As a chief resident traveling between London hospitals, I was pulled over so many times that the police came up with an offer. When you need to move fast, call 999. Explain to the operator and we will take you where you need to go. They did this on several occasions. It wouldn't happen these days. Now they flag me down and I throw a fit. I tell them to check out the incident with the ambulance service, then escort me to the hospital. This conflict pumps up the adrenaline even more. So I'm ready to explode into action. Wield the knife.

The mobile rang at 11:00 p.m. Number "unknown." "Unknown" is always the hospital. The operator said, "I will just connect you with the Accident Department." I was all ears. Pissed off at being disturbed late at night, but listening. The doctor said an ambulance was on its way from Stoke Mandeville Hospital. The patient had a high-velocity gunshot wound to the left chest. He was in shock. Doctors at Stoke Mandeville put him on a drip and said, "Take him directly to Oxford." I asked what turned out to be an Air Force medic how he knew it was high velocity. Because it was a hunting rifle. Was there an exit wound? No. This had important implications for the damage inside. I knew about gunshot wounds. I worked for a time at the Washington Hospital Trauma Center, then at Baraguaneth Township Hospital in Johannesburg. I had written the chapter on "Ballistic Injuries of the Chest" for the military's Emergency Medicine Textbook. I loved operating on penetrating chest wounds. So unpredictable. Every one different. Always a challenge.

"Okay, I'm coming. Could you call my resident? Ask him to call the theater team in." I drove a Jaguar sports car in those days. Before I smashed it to pieces and injured my son. The roads were dark and empty. I could let loose on the accelerator. Keeping a cautious eye for deer or foxes on the road. My mind sifted through the sparse information. How did this guy get shot late in the evening with a high-velocity rifle? High-velocity bullets follow a predictable course but spin rapidly. Had he been shot at shorter range, the bullet would have gone straight out the back of his chest with a larger exit wound. They transfer energy-gouging holes in the lung, generating secondary missiles—fragments of metal, shards of rib, bits of cartilage. Usually fatal.

The unfortunate gentleman lived on the edge of a woodland shooting estate. Just before going to bed, he heard what sounded like gunshots and went out to investigate. It was a full moon, almost Halloween, and cold, with patches of mist in the hollows. He walked down the lane to the edge of the woods and out into the fields. Suddenly, a crashing blow to the chest knocked him off his feet. Even before the sound wave reached him. The crack of rifle fire. There was an agonizing sharp pain above the left nipple. It took his breath away and he felt faint. But kept the presence of mind to use his mobile phone. He dialed 999. Telling the operator he thought he had been shot and providing the location. Then he descended into shock mentally and physically. A moonlit night in the country. He stared up at the stars, fully expecting to die.

His assailant, who happened to be the gamekeeper, was in trouble. He was poaching deer on the property he was supposed to be guarding. He had mistaken the glint of moonlight in the victim's spectacles as a pair of bright eyes. Dropping the rifle sights to a broader target, he pulled the trigger. Aiming at what he expected to be the deer's chest. It was the chest, but not of an animal. And he missed the heart by an inch. A lucky miss. No one survives a high-velocity rifle bullet through the heart. A pistol bullet, yes. Years before at the Middlesex Hospital, I saved a young man shot by the police in East London. The bullet passed straight through his heart but blood clots in the pericardium plugged the holes. This happens when the pressure in the heart falls after blood loss. Not so with high-velocity bullets. They tear the heart to pieces. So I knew our patient didn't have a cardiac injury. I could fix the rest.

I arrived before the patient. The Accident Department was otherwise quiet, so a horde of medical and nursing staff waited to pounce. I needed just one. An anesthetist to insert the tube in his windpipe and secure his breathing. What I didn't want was aggressive fluid infusion to replace the blood loss. Clear fluid raises the blood pressure, promotes bleeding, and impairs the blood's ability to clot. It simply risks catastrophic hemorrhage. Back then, the Advanced Trauma Life Support guidelines were poor, if not dangerous in this respect. Research from Washington, DC, even showed that patients with penetrating chest wounds had better survival when brought to the hospital by private car, rather than by paramedics who spent time putting up drips and pushing in cold fluid.

The ambulance sounded its siren on the approach. By now the patient's blood pressure was less than 60 mm Hg, with a heart rate of 130. He was cold, pale, sweating profusely, and losing consciousness. The paramedics knew that time was running out. They reversed toward the entrance and threw their rear doors open. Down came the ramp and they rushed him into the resuscitation area. I asked him his name, but he didn't respond. He was still wearing the sweaty, bloodstained shirt with a ragged bullet hole in the front. Beneath was the small skin entrance wound, surrounded by a ring of black bruising under pale-white skin. The hole was now plugged by swollen muscle and clotted blood. What's more, I could feel air in the tissues under the skin, a sure sign that the major airways were damaged. I needed to predict the injuries inside from the site of the entry wound. It was not reassuring. The wound was close to the root of the lung. The major clockwork. Over the lung's major blood vessels but away from the heart.

There were far too many cooks about to spoil the broth. I wanted him put to sleep and ventilated quickly so I could cut open his chest and get to the bleeding. He needed a couple of wide-bore venous cannulas in the veins, but there was no time for X-rays or scans. He needed treatment, not investigation. As the anesthetist put the tube down his trachea, I asked the nurses to get me a gown and gloves. Then fetch the chest-opening instruments. Panic spread with the realization that I was about to open him up right there on the trolley. The anesthetic drugs had stolen away what remained of his blood pressure. He was about to arrest. I had to find the bleeding, stop it, then get some donor blood into him. Blood group O can be given to anyone. We keep a stock in the fridge, ready for emergencies. Clear fluid doesn't carry oxygen. Only red cells do that, and he was short of them. I reckoned he had 3 liters or more of blood spilled into the chest cavity. And a collapsed left lung. My resident scrubbed up to join me. I had the nurses roll him onto his side. Left side up. They cut away the wet, bloody shirt with scissors. We rapidly painted the skin with iodine antiseptic. And wiped away the sticky mess. Curiously, I spotted the bullet lying under the skin just beneath the left shoulder blade. It must have been deflected by the scapula bone at the back of the chest, then traveled downward to rest in the center of a bruise. I remember thinking that we should fish it out and keep it for ballistic evidence. To link the bullet with the rifle that fired it.

With a scalpel, I sliced open his chest between the ribs. From the edge of the sternum all the way around to the shoulder blade where the bullet popped out. I kept cutting with the blade. Down through the thick and pale muscle layers. No blood pressure, so there was little left to bleed. As I breached the chest cavity, chunks of clotted blood, liver-like, slithered out and plopped onto the floor. Followed by fresh liquid blood. I grabbed the large rib retractor and cranked open the chest cavity, cracking ribs in my haste. Trying to expose the injuries and visualize the bleeding point. By now, one of my own theater nurses had arrived with a powerful sucker. I could see blood welling up from deep in the depths. As anticipated, the pulmonary artery was lacerated and air was blowing out of the penetrated main bronchial tube. I needed to apply a large clamp across the root of the lung to control both of them. The operating theater nurse scrabbled around trying to find one for me. Once this was safely in place, I told the anesthetist to transfuse him rapidly. The heart was slowing. Grinding to a halt. I could see it right in front of my nose through the thin pericardial sac. I stuck my fist around it and pumped hard for a few cycles. Gave it some help, but it felt empty. I asked for a syringe of adrenaline and stuck the needle directly into the apex of the left ventricle. A couple of milliliters would cheer it up. We needed to get the pressure up and neutralize the lactic acid in his blood with sodium bicarbonate. The adrenaline shot the blood pressure up to acceptable levels, and the heart rate soared up to 140 beats per minute. A fit man, he would bounce back now that we had things under control.

To finish the job properly I needed him under the bright lights of the operating theater. With proper sterile drapes and accurate monitoring of his blood biochemistry and vital signs. By now, it was 2:00 a.m. The theater was ready, the hospital corridors empty. We would wheel him along with his chest wide open. The clamp in place. A drape over the top to keep the wound clean. Then lift him onto the operating table. I threw off my gown and rubber gloves and retrieved the bullet from the floor. Things like that had a habit of disappearing. They become souvenirs. This projectile had great forensic importance. I had to give it to the police, who were accumulating in great numbers. I walked ahead of this bizarre cortege to scrub up again in the operating theater. The nurses were waiting, with the operating lights switched on. Now I could see. I gently removed the clamp, to be met with a gush of dark-blue blood from the pulmonary artery. With the vigorous resuscitation, the chest wound edges were oozing bright-red blood. Air was blowing out of the lacerated bronchial tube. Otherwise, no problem. I pulled on the collapsed, airless lung to get a better view of the damage. It was what you would expect from the high-velocity missile—looking like a dog chewed at the vital structures. My hopes of conserving the lung rapidly dissipated. It had to come out. The whole thing. We needed to make him safe, not attempt some heroic repair job.

If he died, the gamekeeper would face a murder charge. Nor would the family be pleased.

I circled the huge, thin-walled pulmonary artery with a thick silk ligature and gently tied it off. No more dark-blue bleeding. Two large veins enter the heart from the lung. I tied them both off, then cut through all three large blood vessels with scissors. This just left the injured bronchus blowing out blood and froth. I stapled it, chopped through the tube, and lifted out the redundant lung. Like a slippery sponge, it missed the receptacle and fell to the floor. He would be fine with just the one. And the right lung is larger than the left. We washed out the empty space with warm salt solution and the powerful antibiotic gentamicin. Infection was his biggest risk now. The spiraling bullet had sucked fragments of jacket and shirt into the chest.

I sat and wrote notes with drawings while the exhilarated residents stopped bleeding from the wound edges and sewed him up. Documentation is vital in criminal cases. Even at 3:00 a.m. Then my young assistants were eager to talk. So were the police. They didn't get to see many gunshot wounds in sleepy Oxford.

Driving home through the dark lanes, I saw a fox on the grass at the road edge. Then a deer in the headlights. Eyes sparkling. I was relaxed and content. Another battle won. Adrenaline dissipated. Our patient recovered without complications. The gamekeeper was arrested and released on bail. The bullet matched his rifle. He avoided a murder or manslaughter charge by a whisker. Just minutes. Unique case for the "dreaming spires." One for Inspector Morse.

Nothing ignites the adrenaline rush like a stab wound to the heart. I still remember the first one I was dealt as a young man. Way back in 1975. I was what was known as a "casualty officer," working in the Accident Department of Kings College Hospital in South London. On the edge of the war zone that was Brixton, London's equivalent to Harlem, where I encountered many stab wounds. I had already cut my teeth on chests at the Brompton Hospital. Now I was in my "invincible" phase. A coiled spring. Ready to launch into action.

First, some background to set the scene. I really did serve a brief internship in Harlem in New York City, so I knew from experience that most cardiac stab-wound victims die at the site of the incident or on the way to the hospital. Those who do arrive sit on the edge of the precipice. The stakes are high. Most can survive with appropriate treatment. That treatment is immediate surgery. Most assailants attack face to face, stabbing the right ventricle in front. A few wounds involve both right and left ventricles. Stab wounds to the left ventricle usually enter from the flank or back. The "domestic incident" route. The thin-walled right atrium is protected by the breastbone, whereas the left atrium lies further back in the chest. Only rarely are the atria involved in knife wounds.

Rule number one. If the knife or screwdriver is still in place do not remove it. If it is bobbing about with every beat, the blade is likely plugging a hole in the heart muscle. When the patient arrives with the knife in place, it is usually a suicide attempt. Assailants rarely leave their knives and fingerprints as evidence. When a knife is withdrawn, blood under pressure sprays out into the non-distensible pericardial sac. The heart lives in this confined space. If there is free escape of blood out of the pericardium into the expansive chest cavity, this will likely result in exsanguination. The patient bleeds to death. When blood accumulates within the pericardial space because the entry wound is small, we call that "cardiac tamponade." As blood compresses the heart itself, the patient's blood pressure falls. An equilibrium is reached, so the bleeding stops. The circulation is maintained with lower blood pressure. These patients tend to survive. They are brought in pale, cold, and restless with fast heart rate and distended neck veins. But perfectly adequate for survival over a short period of time as long as their blood pressure is kept down.

Rule number two. Those admitted fully conscious usually have cardiac tamponade. Many need immediate chest opening for resuscitation. Holes in the heart are not amenable to standard resuscitation techniques. If given intravenous fluids, such patients will bleed more, often terminally. So it is important to control the bleeding point first. Once the cardiac tamponade is relieved, the patient may not need any fluid. I have operated on tamponade patients who have been given so much fluid that the poor heart was fit to burst. Before sewing the wound, I had to open it up and discard copious amounts of diluted blood into the sucker. Only then did the heart look comfortable enough that I could stitch the laceration.

Some patients arrive still warm but without signs of life. Only if their pupils react to light should emergency surgery be undertaken. With vigorous cardiac massage and adrenaline, I was able to restart any heart. Whether or not the brain was dead. That's why it is important to scrutinize the pupils first. No coroner will allow a murder victim to be kept alive just to be an organ donor.

I wasn't a heart surgeon at Kings. I was still a junior doctor. It was 2:00 a.m. The department was full of drug addicts, drunks, vagrants, and the walking wounded. Not that we didn't care for them. We did. The nurses were saints but constantly needed protection. It was a volatile environment. This particular patient was dumped in the entrance hall by fellow gang members. His shirt covered in blood. Ashen and already unconscious. The porters brought him through to a resuscitation bay, and the sister in charge called the resuscitation team. He still had a faint pulse, and his pupils reacted to light. As the nurses removed his shirt, I could see the stab wound directly over the heart. Around 1 centimeter in width. Blood trickled from the edges, but it wasn't pumping. The jugular veins stood out like tree trunks in his skinny neck because of raised pressure within the pericardial sac. This was obviously cardiac tamponade. The anesthetist had already inserted the endotracheal tube and was frantically ventilating the lungs. We still needed a large-bore cannula in a neck vein for transfusion. A nurse took over, squeezing the gas bag while the anesthetist did the deed. He couldn't miss. Dark-blue blood shot out the end at high pressure.

In those days, there were no senior medics in the emergency room at night. Certainly no cardiac surgeons in the hospital. The sister knew I had worked at the Brompton. She just looked at me and said, "Open him up. I will help you." The anesthetist was a senior resident. He nodded in approval, well aware that the kid would die if we did nothing. External cardiac massage is futile when the heart is compressed and cannot fill. There wasn't even time to scrub up. The assembled crowd rolled him over left side up while I pulled on a gown and gloves. Sister followed suit. He had no pulse or blood pressure. I stood behind him. Sister in front. With my own adrenaline pumping, I carved the chest open with a scalpel. Then spread the ribs with a metal retractor stored ready for this eventuality but rarely used. There was no blood or air in the chest cavity. The stiletto knife had gone directly through the front of the pericardium into the right ventricle. All I could see was the tense, blue, bulging pericardial sac. I knew what I had to do. If I could stop my own perspiration from clouding my eyes and dripping into the incision.

I opened the stretched fibrous membrane with a scalpel. Blood and blood clot spewed out. The heart was still beating, but empty. The ventricles filled as the pericardium emptied. His blood pressure started to come up and the stab wound started to squirt out blood again. Not an issue now. I put my index finger over the gash. I said, "Transfuse him while I stitch the ventricle." Sister asked, "What stitch do you want?" I didn't have any idea. I just said, "Give me anything you've got on a curved needle." The first needle was much too big. The next much too small. But the third was just right. A blue-colored braided suture that knotted well. Perfect. I swapped fingers with Sister, who had never touched a heart before. She was squirted with blood as we swapped over. Now the tricky bit. I mounted the curved needle on the needle holder and edged into the best position to throw the stitch. I knew that as soon as Sister moved her finger, blood would be pissing out. Not only that. The young heart was now bounding away. A rapidly moving target. Not easy to stitch accurately. Deep breath. Just get on and do it. I drove the needle straight through the middle of the laceration. From one side to the other. With deep bites. Sister cut the needle from the suture material and I gently tied the knot. It worked, but to make him safe, I needed another stitch on either side. Three in total. Nerve-wracking for an amateur. Each time the needle penetrated the muscle, it triggered a run of fast, uncontrolled rhythm. I'd guess all three stitches took me ten minutes. Today I could do it in less than two.

Sister looked straight at me over her mask. She was impressed. Actually, so was I. The hero of the moment. The blood pressure and heart rate were soon normal. Just when we no longer needed him, the cardiothoracic resident had been called in. By now I was happy to leave him to it. Sister and I retired to the coffee room. Sweaty but elated. With the chest closed up, they rolled him onto his back on the trolley. There was blood everywhere. On the stretcher canvas, in his hair, soaking his clothes, and drying in a pool on the floor. Testament to our struggle. They needed to get him to the ICU for a cleanup. By now there were scores of other patients in the department. All growing restless with the wait. Then the patient suddenly woke up, uncontrollably agitated following the near-death experience. He sat bolt upright and began tugging at the IVs. The jugular vein cannula in the neck disconnected. As he took a deep breath in, negative pressure in his chest sucked air into the circulation and he collapsed. Pulseless again for a different reason. At the time no one realized why it had happened. They started external cardiac massage but couldn't revive him. My first solo heart operation had proved fatal. From hero to zero. Shit and derision.

Suddenly the night turned into a nightmare. Paranoia set in. I was concerned that I would be blamed for the death. Accused of recklessness. I shouldn't have worried. Sister and the anesthetist made clear the situation. Without my intervention, he would have been dead sooner. The case went to the coroner's court. The verdict? Unlawful killing. The cause of death? Air embolism after a cardiac stab wound. Not only was this my debut emergency thoracotomy, it was my first encounter with this fatal complication. Air reaching the vessels of the brain. Sadly, it was not the last. I was destined to operate on many more cardiac stab wounds throughout my career. Most simple. Some complex, involving the heart valves or coronary arteries. None of them died.

Knives and bullets are not the only sources of penetrating chest wounds. Some of the most horrifically violent injuries occur during road-traffic accidents. It was 2005. One quiet Saturday afternoon in autumn, I was waiting for my son's rugby to start. The mobile rang and I was required to scramble again. For an immediately life-threatening injury in a young woman. Mark's school was ten minutes from the hospital. I was waiting in the hospital before the unfortunate victim arrived. Input from the paramedics en route suggested that a car had veered off the A40 divided highway at high speed, shattering a wooden fence. A sharp shard of wood the size of a spear had penetrated the windshield and transfixed the driver's neck. The fire brigade had extricated her from the wreck, but she was blowing air from the wound and had difficulty breathing. Her blood pressure was low, so they suspected internal bleeding.

The trauma team was waiting in the resuscitation area—but warning lights were flashing in my brain. It sounded as if her windpipe was cut in two. If so, blind attempts to pass the breathing tube could push the ends apart and completely obstruct the airway. I wanted an experienced cardiothoracic anesthetist to join us. And the cardiac operating-theater team to stand by. I called Dr. Mike Sinclair myself. Asked him to come at top speed, which he did. As we waited, I politely requested that the resuscitation team should hold off until I had the chance to examine the girl. It was already more than an hour since the crash. If she was still alive, it meant that she had reached some degree of equilibrium. A couple of minutes to work out the likely injuries would be time well spent.

Tension rose palpably as the girl was wheeled in. She was awake, but deathly pale. Rigid with fear. Blue lips. All eyes were immediately drawn to the gash at the root of her neck on the right side. Bare sternomastoid muscle was exposed while air raised the torn skin as she exhaled. It sounded as if she were farting through her wound with every breath. And spraying an aerosol of blood. I had no doubt about the cause. Equally, I was incredulous that the transfixion hadn't ripped out at least one of her two carotid arteries. If so, she would have died at the scene.

She feebly raised her right arm. Inviting me to take her sweaty hand. I was pleased to do that. Instinctively, I told her she would be fine. Not that I knew it, but she needed some comfort. To be treated like a person, not an object of curiosity. Now I needed the poor girl's clothes off. She was in shock. Not just mental distress. She had clearly lost liters of blood internally. My guess was that the stake had passed downward through the neck and into the left chest, taking out a significant blood vessel. A good old stethoscope would tell me that. Physical examination was quick and still important in this era of fancy scans. Air was still filling the right lung, but there were no breath sounds on the left. When I tapped the ribs, the left chest was "dull to percussion." An old-fashioned physical sign of fluid surrounding the lung. So she had blood in the chest and barely recordable blood pressure. Heart rate, 110 beats per minute. Now we had a surgical conundrum. A severe injury to the root of the neck, together with bleeding into the left chest. A tricky combination. Yet the basic principles remained the same. First establish a safe and reliable airway. Next, take control of the breathing. Then support the circulation. In this case by stopping the bleeding and blood transfusion. The ABC of resuscitation.

I needed Mike to put her to sleep. The only reliable way to secure her airway was with an old-fashioned rigid bronchoscope. We had done hundreds of bronchoscopies together. To investigate lung cancer or to remove inhaled peanuts from children. By now the resuscitation team had put a couple of drips in her arms and were giving clear fluids. I didn't want too much of that. She was critical but stable. The same old story. Then Mike walked in and we agreed to push her directly over to the operating theaters. There I had ultimate control, surrounded by my own team. Away from the circus.

Sister Linda had the bronchoscope prepared and waiting in the anesthetic room. Mike needed to anesthetize and paralyze her. Then I could slip this rigid brass telescope through the back of her throat, through her vocal cords, and into the injured trachea. High-pressure ventilation through the scope sprayed blood out of her neck. But I could soon see the injury. Two-thirds of the circumference of the trachea was lacerated. Only the muscular back wall was intact. I pushed a long, stiff rubber probe down the bronchoscope and through the site of injury. After vigorously blowing in air to raise her oxygen levels, the bronchoscope was withdrawn. Mike could then railroad his breathing tube safely over this guide. "A" and "B" sorted. We could ventilate the lungs safely. Now I had to get on and stop the life-threatening bleeding. They wheeled her through into the operating theater and turned her so she was left side up. Scrub nurse Pauline was already scrubbed up and had laid out the thoracotomy instruments on sterile linen. I didn't have to say a word. It all just happened around me. Like clockwork. Mike was ready with two units of donor blood. He now had arterial blood pressure monitoring on the screen via a cannula in the wrist.

A range of thoughts went through my mind at the scrub sink. First, I was relieved for the poor woman that she was unconscious. Remote from her terrifying ordeal. Then I was uncharacteristically apprehensive. What would I find in the apex of the chest? I feared laceration of the large subclavian artery to her arm, difficult to access, though she still had a pulse at the left wrist. I hoped it was just low-pressure venous bleeding. Easier to control. I was cognizant of the fact that the nerves to the arm were close by. I needed to avoid damage to them with the electrocautery.

Two liters of blood spilled out of the chest. Splashing onto the floor over my trousers and clogs. Warm and wet. Wasted. With compression relieved, the left lung expanded like a kid's balloon. Virginal pink. Not like the mottled gray lungs of smokers. We scooped and sucked blood from the depths of the chest until the ragged hole came into view. Mercifully, there was no bright-red arterial hemorrhage. Just dark-red bleeding from the main arm vein. I set about stopping the bleeding. If I tied off the vein, her arm would swell. So I clamped and repaired it with a patch from a less important vein to preserve the flow. Now I was content that she was safe. We washed the chest cavity out with antiseptic solution. All the other main arteries and nerves were clearly visible in the roof of the chest. The stake had simply pushed them aside. Generously limited its destruction to the least important structures. The luck of the girl was barely credible. "C" for "circulation" was now sorted. We were left with one other major injury to sort out. The transected trachea. A big tube containing air. Much less intimidating. We closed up the chest, leaving a drain to remove residual air and blood. I injected a generous volume of long-acting local anesthetic into the nerves under the ribs to dull the pain. She had suffered enough.

It was time for a cup of tea while they rolled her onto her back. By now I was relaxed, ready to explore the neck wound. I liked to operate in the neck. Hers was slender with no fat, making everything easier. The horrendous gash was 10 centimeters in length, just above the joint between the sternum and clavicle, gaping widely to reveal bare muscle. Like grinning lips exposing teeth. The simplest approach was to excise the ragged wound edges, then extend the cut to the left into a thyroid gland incision. Her lacerated trachea was right in front of me. The thyroid gland above. The rigid plastic breathing tube passing through the gap. With the benefit of full resuscitation, the wound edges oozed bright-red blood. Easy to stop. Because the rural fence post was likely covered with bacteria, I excised the contaminated edges of the trachea, and then joined the clean ends with multiple separate sutures. All of which was an intimidating problem but easy surgery. I managed a solid airtight repair and finished by checking the nerves to the vocal cords. Again these were spared what might have been. God must have been with her in the car. Or sitting on my shoulder. Maybe both. Mike gave her a slug of heavy-duty antibiotics for good measure. Finally, we closed the skin and subcutaneous layers with metal clips. Job well done.

The family was huddled anxiously in the ICU. They had come in through the Accident Department, inoculated with a dose of pessimism and then dispatched for the long wait. Waiting to be told the outcome of emergency surgery is a truly miserable experience. When it's your own kid and they tell you that a fence post nearly took her head off. Alive or dead? Disabled or intact? Disfigured or still beautiful? Difficult to concentrate on Saturday's sports results. I told them what I told her. When I squeezed her hand as life ebbed away. That everything would be okay. Then I rode off into the sunset. As far as the pub, that is. For time with my own little family. To hear about my son's rugby and my daughter's golf match. The fights. The cuts and the bruises. And that was just the ladies' golf.

Everything really was okay. She recovered quickly. Mike and I came in on Sunday morning. She was wide awake, so we pulled out the tracheal tube. Inevitably, she felt like she had been hit by a truck. Her throat and chest were sore. But her breathing was fine and she could speak. Everything was intact—and she went home in a week.

Thankfully, with age my adrenaline addiction and testosterone are wearing off, yet the excitement of the unexpected persists. For the unfortunate patient, any prospect of survival depends on having an experienced trauma surgeon at hand. Few are afforded that privilege. Then you might ask, "What does he know about spitfire pilots?" Perhaps more than you imagine. My father-in-law fought the Battle of Britain. He was "one of the few," as Churchill described them. A true hero. Not a cardboard cutout like me!

fourteen Despair

Strength does not come from winning.
Your struggles develop your strengths. When you go through
hardships and decide not to surrender, that is strength.

—Arnold Schwarzenegger

OXFORD BROOKES UNIVERSITY IS WITHIN ONE MILE OF MY hospital. It is full of vibrant, happy students. One of them, a twenty-year-old girl studying Japanese language, had complained of fainting attacks. A series of preliminary investigations including an ECG and echocardiogram indicated that her heart was normal. One evening when she was talking with friends on the campus, she suddenly collapsed to the floor. This was only a few days after the public resuscitation of a premier-league soccer player on the field in London, an event widely covered on the television. He survived through effective bystander resuscitation by a cardiologist on the grounds. Then rapid transport to a front-line cardiac center. As a result, cardiopulmonary resuscitation was very much in the public awareness. The girl's friends began cardiac massage and called the emergency services. A paramedic ambulance was dispatched from the nearby headquarters and reached her in less than four minutes.

Their cardiac monitor showed ventricular fibrillation—the heart squirming aimlessly, not pumping. These days, all paramedic vehicles carry a defibrillator. As the girl's friends continued chest compressions, the paramedics set up to defibrillate. They put the electrodes on the front and left side of her chest. Ninety joules. Zap. This usually works in heart-attack patients, but after a brief period of flatline it fibrillated again. The hospital was two minutes away. Less than a mile. Full of specialist doctors. But they didn't bring her in. They inserted a tube into the windpipe and persisted with on-site resuscitation. At least she was getting oxygen.

The ambulance was carrying a new toy. A "Lucas" chest-compression machine. Manual cardiac massage is tiring, but the machine doesn't tire. It rhythmically pushes down on the lower half of the breastbone, forcing blood out of the heart and around the body. When more shocks failed, they fitted the machine around her chest. Now her heart was squeezed between the sternum and spine. Continuously pounded like a meat tenderizer. Time passed. It was more than thirty minutes after the cardiac arrest that she was wheeled in to the Accident Department. Lifeless, but replete with medical equipment. Lucas machine still bashing away. Her pupils still reacting to light. They must be congratulated for keeping her brain alive. Yet the poor heart was still squirming. Battered and bruised.

The soccer player was lucky. There was an experienced cardiologist right there on the grounds. What this young woman needed was treatment targeted toward the underlying problem. What she got was the Standard Advanced Life Support approach. First defibrillation, using increasingly higher voltage. Repeated failure. Persistent fibrillation. Continuous cardiac compression by the machine. Then adrenaline injected into a vein. Potentially useful when the heart is contracting, but this worsens muscle irritability and predisposes it to more ventricular fibrillation. Then she was given the drug amiodarone in an attempt to calm the electrical storm. Good move, but after thirty shocks she still reverted back to ventricular fibrillation.

With the situation looking desperate, the on-call cardiologist, Dr. Bashir, arrived. Fortunately, he was an experienced electrophysiologist. He looked carefully at the patient and changed the position of the electrodes on the chest. He placed one on the front of the chest, over the right ventricle, and one on her back, directly behind the left ventricle. With one shock of 200 joules, normal heart rhythm was restored. With adrenaline on board, the blood pressure immediately rose to above-normal levels. This had the benefit of increasing blood flow to the traumatized heart muscle but also increased electrical instability. The result? Repeated fibrillation. This needed more shocks and a high dose of beta blocker to counter the stimulant. With the electrodes in better position, the shocks worked each time. Dr. Bashir then prescribed a combination of powerful rhythm-stabilizing drugs in high doses.

Around two hours after the first collapse, the erratic rhythm began to settle. She became stable enough for an echo study to obtain pictures of the heart. Whatever this showed would be revealing. Only a handful of problems caused sudden death in young people. One of the possibilities was an inherited condition with thick heart muscle. The echo soon ruled that out. Both ventricles were normal in size and thickness. By now the right ventricle directly beneath the sternum was suffering visibly after prolonged cardiac massage and electric shocks. It was dilated and contracting poorly. The heart valves all appeared normal. Very rare coronary artery abnormalities can cause ventricular fibrillation. What could be seen of these small vessels also appeared normal. This was electrical instability in a structurally normal, now battered little heart. A primary ventricular dysrhythmia. This can present as fainting attacks or sudden cardiac death without any identifiable genetic syndrome, not related to exercise or stress but probably arising from within the heart's own electrical system. It can happen in short bursts of electrical instability or as a full blown "electrical storm." If it settled, it could be treated by electrical mapping to locate the origin, and then followed by destruction of the irritable source. This was Dr. Bashir's specialty, performed in the catheter laboratory. It can also be done during the electrical storm if the patient's circulation can be sustained in the meantime. This is not easy to organize at night, as it requires a highly trained support team.

The plan was to move her from the Accident Department to the cardiac ICU. Senior intensive care doctors were already involved. Working to normalize her blood chemistry after three hours of resuscitation. They were already anxious that she was sliding into heart failure. They wanted my opinion as to whether she would need mechanical circulatory support.

I arrived at the Accident Department at 9:30 p.m. There was a crowd around her bed in the resuscitation area. Most of them doing nothing. Spectators. The cardiac massage machine was still in place. Thankfully, it had been switched off while her rhythm was normal. Personally, I disliked it. Cardiac massage is vitally important, but the heart is a delicate organ. It needs just the right pressure. I don't like it to be palped by a machine. By now the intensive-care doctors had her well sedated and ventilated. The blood chemistry had improved because normal rhythm had given her better blood flow. The cardiology resident lingered nervously by the defibrillator. I had only been there three minutes when she fibrillated again. This time, no pounding on the chest. Finger on the trigger. Zap and back to sinus rhythm. I suggested that we take her directly to the ICU. Get the sledgehammer back into the ambulance, away from the broken ribs. After seventy electrical shocks, we settled on the diagnosis of idiopathic ventricular fibrillation. Her heart was beginning to respond to the anti-dysrhythmic drugs. Perhaps it was wise not to move her to the catheter laboratory at this stage—while we appeared to be winning. The shocks became less frequent, the heart easier to defibrillate.

We stayed with her in the ICU. Right by the bedside. During the night, her parents and boyfriend arrived after a terrible journey from the North. Poleaxed with grief and anxiety. I was watching as the nurses told them the story. Then the look on their faces when they first saw her in the bed. On the ventilator, pale with blue lips, big drips in the neck, arms, and wrist. How intensive care always looks, but a terrible shock the first time. Even more terrible when it's your child hovering between life and death. Then the quiet descent into recrimination. How could this have happened? She seemed so happy at Brookes. Did she get it from us? This was the time to ask her parents about the medical history. I asked my resident to do it. I couldn't face it. I hovered in the background. Had anyone in the family died suddenly? Was there any history of heart disease? Had she had problems before? Each drew a blank.

I knew what to expect. It was why I stayed. Hoping that it wouldn't happen. When the adrenaline wore off, the electrical irritability lessened but the blood pressure started to creep down. By the early morning, it was worryingly low. Meanwhile, the pressure in the veins drifted upward as the right ventricle struggled to cope. Battered, bruised, now sliding down inexorably. Acid in the blood started to rise, produced by the muscles as their blood flow dwindled. She needed more shocks in front of her parents. There was no time to usher them away. A grim reminder to them that she was actually dying. Her hands and legs were cold with the onset of cardiogenic shock—shock not from the dysrhythmia but from the heavy-duty cardiac massage and repeated electrical trauma. And not helped by the high-dose beta blocker we needed to counteract the adrenaline.

I asked for another echo. This time taken through a probe in the gullet. The camera sits right behind the heart so the pictures are much better. Things had changed dramatically for the worse. Both the left and right ventricles were contracting poorly. This is when the "what ifs" kick in. Would this have happened if the defibrillating electrodes had been positioned differently? What if they had rushed her straight into the hospital? Then she could have been treated sooner by those who could make the diagnosis and target the drug treatment, as my colleague had done. It needed expertise and drugs. Not a mechanical sledgehammer out in the town.

"What ifs" are no good in cardiac surgery. We have to get on and treat what lies in front of us. I knew what she needed now. The struggling heart was still recoverable, but she needed circulatory support. The only thing we could do quickly was to insert an intra-aortic balloon pump. Well aware that it was nearly useless in shocked patients. It went in anyway and slightly improved the blood pressure on the monitor. But she needed more blood flow and the balloon doesn't provide that. We had to start the vasopressor drug noradrenaline to keep the pressure above 70 mm Hg. Soon that triggered further episodes of ventricular fibrillation. She needed a ventricular assist device to take over the circulation, like the pumps we had before the charitable money ran out. Our patient had both left and right ventricular failure and her lungs were deteriorating in response to the shock. In this case we needed a system called extra-corporeal membrane oxygenation, or ECMO, for short. This combines a centrifugal blood pump with an oxygenator. It's similar to the oxygenator in the heart-lung machine but engineered for long-term use, safe for days or weeks until the heart gets better. But we didn't have it. Only a handful of UK hospitals were funded to use it, primarily for patients with severe lung disease. By now my own blood was beginning to boil: As I watched the despairing parents by the bedside. As I watched the watery spring sun peep over the horizon. As normal healthy people were beginning their day. Just as she did yesterday at Oxford Brookes.

So what did the recent National Institute for Health and Clinical Excellence (NICE) guidelines for Acute Heart Failure have to say? They glibly suggested to "ask advice from a hospital that has circulatory support equipment." Really helpful, so we did. My surgical colleagues whom I had trained said she needed ECMO. What were the prospects for safe transfer of a dying girl who was suffering ventricular fibrillation at regular intervals? Who had been shocked seventy times. Whose heart was battered. The odds of getting her to another center in safety were negligible. No one disputed that fact. My colleagues in the transplant center expressed surprise that we had no ECMO system, given our track record of innovation. I simply had to get the equipment brought to Oxford by the company representative. As soon as possible. Much like my efforts with the Berlin Heart. We couldn't locate the supplier until 8:30 a.m. By then the blood pressure had sagged again, with a rise in pressure in the veins. As a result the tissues were poorly perfused. Blood flow within the vital organs was critically impaired. I debated whether to take her to the operating theater and put her on a conventional heart-lung machine. Yet this could have been a disaster for a number of reasons. The inflammatory response would further damage the lungs and the ability of the blood to clot. Bleeding is the most common life-threatening complication during ECMO. After prolonged standard cardiopulmonary bypass, the risks would be even greater. There was one other temporizing option—a powerful heart-failure drug called Levosimendan that we had used successfully in the past. It helps link calcium to the muscle molecules and increases the force of contraction. And it does so without increasing tissue oxygen uptake or ventricular irritability. I asked the intensive-care doctors to start an infusion of the drug. Only to be told that we didn't stock it anymore. It was apparently too expensive. All we had were drugs to constrict the blood vessels and make the heart more irritable. Drugs that would flog her struggling heart and make things worse.

We were desperately trying to keep this young woman alive without the equipment or the drugs she needed. It was a tense and miserable morning watching the clock tick away. Trying to reassure the parents that we were doing everything we could. Waiting for the ECMO equipment. Infusing vials of sodium bicarbonate to neutralize the acid. Watching her pupils. Did they still react to light? Was the brain getting enough oxygen? Higher doses of arterial constrictor drugs would briefly elevate the blood pressure, and possibly increase flow to the brain but at the expense of her limbs and gut. Her hands and legs were already cold and white. This was critically low blood flow with acid pouring into the circulation from muscles starved of oxygen.

By midday I couldn't watch any longer. I went around to the operating theaters and told them that we had no choice but to put her on cardiopulmonary bypass. I hoped just for a short time, until the ECMO equipment reached the hospital. Then someone asked the inevitable. Who was going to pay for ECMO? Who was going to look after it at night? What if? I was tired and irritable. So I let rip. Who were they to question our efforts to save a twenty-year-old? So what if we weren't a transplant center? She didn't need a transplant. Her own heart needed a rest from the battering of the last twenty-four hours. Something we had done many times before but without NHS funding. Why was this so-called center of excellence unable to save a kid who had collapsed within a mile of the hospital? It certainly wasn't through lack of effort by the medical staff. Just as I was about to lose it altogether, I heard that the equipment had arrived. She was already on the way to the theater, so I went to meet the company representative who had made an enormous effort to help us. He had been in Oxford for more than an hour. Stuck in traffic trying to get into the hospital. Then driving around in circles to find a parking space. Lost time. Lower chance of survival. He knew it and was extremely pissed off.

Once the equipment was ready it took us just minutes to establish the ECMO circuit via an artery and vein in each groin. Ultrasounds of the femoral blood vessels showed the artery to be narrow. Because of this, I chose to surgically expose it and join a vascular graft to the side. This would guarantee that the leg still received adequate blood flow. The femoral vein in the opposite groin was cannulated directly, using a needle and guidewire. The long cannula was advanced into the right atrium and positioned carefully, using an echo probe in the esophagus. When the pump was turned on, the blood pressure immediately rose to 110/70 mm Hg. The pressure in the veins fell from 25 mm Hg to 5 mm Hg. She was transformed by the ECMO system within a few minutes. Better color, better chemistry, different patient. I was jubilant. The parents relaxed.

For the first few hours, her pupils remained responsive to light. Then late in the afternoon when the heart had improved substantially, the pupils suddenly dilated widely and became unreactive to light. My nightmare scenario. Body better. Brain busted. Starved of blood and oxygen, it had started to swell. The pressure within the bony confines of the skull went up and the brain stem herniated into the spinal canal. Medical jargon for fucking disaster.

At the time, I was lying on the sofa in my office. Hoping that the battle was over. Sue knocked tentatively on the door before heading for home. The ICU had asked that I go back, a message that always gives me that sinking feeling. No one calls with good news. Always trouble. I expected bleeding. Something that I could sort out. When I reached the bed space, the curtains were pulled around. Her parents were seated on either side, each holding a hand. Now drained both physically and emotionally. I needed to know what the issues were before I disturbed them. The distraught nurse looking after her came out to talk. Her patient's pupils had blown quite quickly. I needed to know the cause. Whether she had intra-cerebral bleeding from the heparin anticoagulation or a swollen brain through lack of oxygen. A brain surgeon might be able to help with the first. By removing the blood clot. The second was more than likely to signal a fatal conclusion to our efforts. Just when we had beaten off the ventricular fibrillation. It was four hours since the last shock. Now we needed to go to the brain scanner as soon as possible. I went to arrange it myself. And asked a brain surgeon colleague to come and look at it with me.

Brain scans emerge slice by slice, multiple cross sections through convoluted gray and white matter. This is complex but well-charted anatomy, each part responsible for part of our lives. Yet some parts are more important than others. The skull is a rigid box. When the brain swells, something has to give. The fluid spaces are compressed and disappear. The delicate brain appendages and nerves are distorted. Eventually parts of the brain stem are pushed out of the skull. Hence the loss of the pupils' reaction to light. And when brain stem reflexes are lost, the patient is dead. The whole scan of the girl's brain was finished in minutes. Then the slices were computed into a three-dimensional reconstruction of the entire organ. It told a story I didn't want to read. "Severe brain swelling with herniation of brain stem through the foramen magnum" was the official radiologist's report. I tried to persuade the brain surgeons to decompress the brain. They were sympathetic but said it was too late. Sorry about that. But not as sorry as I was. We pushed her back to the ICU. Quite an undertaking in itself with all the equipment—ECMO circuit, ventilator, balloon pump, monitoring equipment. Moved now in a sad procession.

What were we left with? All her other organs were recovering. She was warm and pink. Flooded with well-oxygenated blood from the lifesaving equipment that came too late. Kidneys making urine. Gut absorbing feed. Liver removing toxins. All organs need blood and oxygen. This simple, inexpensive technology supplied both with abundance. But too late for the brain. The cells that we failed to save were the cells that matter most. I was bitter about this. No other team in the United Kingdom had our breadth of pioneering experience. We had put in the hard graft in the laboratory, had made the important discoveries. We had done all that for the first time. But that didn't matter to the authorities. What mattered was that we weren't a transplant center and were therefore not eligible for funding. Only a handful of hospitals are allowed the equipment to rescue those with severe heart failure. What matters in the NHS is keeping down costs. Death is cheap.

I couldn't face telling her parents. I took the coward's way out and went back to my office. Black as thunder. The intensive-care doctors did their best to treat the brain swelling with drugs. Going through the motions. But the die was cast. ECMO was withdrawn after forty-eight hours because of brain death. I took the tubes out myself. By now her heart was working well. Good blood pressure, normal rhythm, no ventricular fibrillation. Too late.

After formal tests for brain stem death, the issue of organ donation was raised with the grieving mom and dad. Apparently, she had previously expressed the wish to donate her organs in the event of premature death. The family agreed. Before this, I went to see her while the parents were still there. So was the nurse who had helped us battle for her life. She wanted to stay to the bitter end. To see it through and support them. Uncommon decency, and that takes moral fiber and courage. What could I say at this point? I was desperately sad. My son was a fellow Brookes student of similar age. How would I have felt in their shoes? I didn't have to think about that. I had faced so many bereaved parents that I knew. What I told them was this: I was deeply sorry for their loss. Given the difficult circumstances, an experienced team of senior medics had fought day and night to turn things around. All of my colleagues were devastated by the outcome. We appreciated the kind offer to donate her organs. It was a gesture that would transform the lives of others. In the end, she donated her liver and kidneys so three patients benefited. The fact that these organs still functioned normally was a testament to ECMO.

Within days, we needed the ECMO apparatus again. This time for a young woman who had just given birth and suffered an embolism of uterine fluid to her lungs. All I could advise was to send her directly to an ECMO center. So I did my duty by NICE. Participated in the cost containment. I knew full well that the delay would prove fatal. It did. Leaving the newborn infant without a mother. Then I could have used it for a forty-year-old patient who suffered accidental air embolism and cardiac arrest in our own ICU. She died. And so the list of lives unnecessarily cut short goes on. And on. Without charity, I am not in the position to save people.

My patient's death caused real distress among her university friends and teachers. So much so that I wrote to the vice chancellor, to express my own regret that we couldn't save her after her friends had made such a valiant effort when she collapsed. Months later, I received an invitation to the Oxford Brookes graduation ceremony. They intended to award her a posthumous degree and would I please come with the parents. I sat with her mom, dad, and boyfriend in the front row. We watched the bright young men and women come up to the stage to collect their awards. Happy and successful. Then the chancellor, Shami Chakrabarti, gave the explanation about the special award and thanked the surgeon for his valiant attempts to save her. Someone had to go up and receive the certificate. Mom was the one. Dad was frozen with grief. Her boyfriend sat desolate. I was choked. I couldn't speak, but I helped the poor mother stumble up the stairs. This was not how it was meant to be. Not the anticipated end to her university career. All her friends and tutors rallied round. The family was happy to see them. Bravely, they went to the reception. I went away crushed, the weight of the world on my shoulders. The saddest day of my whole career.

In memory of Alice Hunter—so that others might live.

fifteen   Double Jeopardy

When I was young and full of life,
I loved the local doctor's wife,
And ate an apple every day,
To keep the doctor far away.

—Thomas W. Lamont

JULIA WAS FORTY. PRETTY, BLONDE, AND FEISTY, WITH A busy career in London. On weekends, she was an accomplished event rider, not far from the top tier, rubbing shoulders, or bridle, with the best. So she had left that competition late to have her first baby. It would be fine. She was fit, physically and mentally. As a psychology student at Durham University, she had played hockey for the university, then for her county, Leicestershire. And soccer. And cricket. One funny thing. Despite all that, she could never complete a high-intensity exercise test. Something always held her back. And she fell asleep in meetings. Regularly and reproducibly. So much so that she was admitted to a private hospital for sleep studies. They suspected narcolepsy. Nothing was found, but it cost a bit.

She was deliriously excited when the pregnancy test turned blue. April 2015. Only the second month of trying. Bingo. Then she started to get really tired. Then a bit breathless. Then more breathless—just getting onto the horse. They reassured her that it was normal in pregnancy. It was down to hormones and retained fluid. Desperate not to let this beat her, she started running again. Determined to get fitter. The first time, she pushed herself for 5 kilometers. The next week, she was breathless by the end of the street, and with a burning throat and tight chest. Her breasts were tender and swollen. Julia thought sore breasts could be part of the problem. She had to slow down a bit. But she could still ride. At thirteen weeks, she saw the midwife at the doctor's office. On a Monday. She was advised to take aspirin as prophylaxis against pre-eclampsia—the dangerously high blood pressure some women suffer during the later stages of pregnancy. She mentioned how unfit she felt, how quickly the situation had deteriorated. Instead of dismissing Julia as neurotic, the midwife's response was, "Let's get your heart and lungs checked out. I'll have a word with the doctor." The midwife's decision to act turned out to be critically important.

The doctor was kind and reassuring. "Blood volume increases by a third during pregnancy. It can make you breathless. Let me listen to your chest." Then the tone changed. He looked serious now. "Just a slight murmur. But we should get you seen quickly." Soon he was on the phone to the private Windsor Clinic in Maidenhead. A cardiologist would see her on Wednesday, the day after tomorrow. Julia was anxious but went back to work. United Biscuits needed her, and working would keep her mind off the "murmur" word.

The Windsor Clinic had a nice waiting room, an efficient receptionist, and a comfortable sofa. None of which mattered a whit to Julia. There were two important tests planned before she saw the cardiologist. Off with the smart black dress, on with the papery white gown with ties down the back. First, the electrocardiogram. So up on the exam table and off with the top of the gown. Electrodes on wrists, ankles, and across the chest wall. The ECG machine rapidly spewed out a long strip of pink paper with a black squiggly line. Crucial to doctors. Meaningless to anyone else. The technician said it was fine. How reassuring. Except it wasn't fine. To the tutored eye, Julia's ECG showed what we call left ventricular hypertrophy. Heart muscle under strain. Next, an echocardiogram. The non-invasive window on the heart. Ultrasound pictures, taken with a probe and projected on a screen. This time by a male tech. Julia blushed a bit. Nice man. Chatty as he smeared the viscous jelly on her chest. All part of the job.

It took a while to get good pictures. Working around the swollen left breast. Trying not to hurt. First the heart chambers. Left and right ventricle. Seen best through the "four chamber" view. The left ventricle was thicker than expected. Right ventricle, left atrium, and right atrium all normal. The technician shifted the probe to the top of the breastbone, angled it downward. Then his demeanor and expression changed. He went quiet and fiddled with the probe. Julia sensed impending bad news. That sudden cold, empty feeling. Like your guts just fell out. "What is it?" she asked involuntarily. "Tight aortic stenosis," came an automatic reply. "I'm so sorry. I will go and tell the doctor." Then another lady came with a different echo machine to look for the baby. Slimy jelly on the belly. This was Julia's first introduction to her fetus. It was important to establish that it was still alive. Then from the dialogue a sense that it might be better if it wasn't. While Julia's day was unraveling, the fetal heart was still beating away normally. Around 150 beats per minute.

It was time to see the doctor, a smart young cardiologist who also worked in the NHS. He had already reviewed her workup. He knew the diagnosis, but there was nothing he could do to help. At least she had her clothes on now. Julia felt less exposed, less physically vulnerable but verging on psychological meltdown. Although she knew about psychology, it didn't make it easier to control her own. She spoke first. No pleasantries. "I'm in trouble, aren't I?"

"Yes, I'm sorry." That bloody word again. All doctors use it. Nobody means it.

"You have severe aortic stenosis. Congenital aortic stenosis. Didn't anyone hear the murmur before you decided to have the child?" Julia thought carefully. Other doctors had listened to her chest. But no. No one had mentioned a heart murmur. When the valve becomes tight, it can be difficult to hear one. Now it was very tight, those symptoms unveiled by the expanded blood volume, by the extra work that a heart has to do to support the placenta.

From the twelfth to the thirty-sixth week of gestation, the volume of blood pumped by the heart rises to a peak of 50 percent above non-pregnant levels. Julia had hit the buffers by thirteen weeks, because she had a severe narrowing of the valve at the outlet of the left ventricle. The crushing chest pain when she exercised stemmed from poor flow in the coronary arteries. When the pressure in her arm was 100 mm Hg, that in her left ventricle was 250 mm Hg. Dangerously high. And blood trying to enter the heart was held back in the lungs, causing them to be stiff. Further strain of any kind could cause edema fluid to flood the lungs, risking sudden death. And Julia thought she was fit!

Now the coup de grâce. The life expectancy for severe aortic stenosis without the baby would be between six to twenty-four months at best. In Julia's current situation, it was weeks. It was far too dangerous to continue with the pregnancy. The cardiologist felt that he should arrange an abortion before the weekend. Then it would be possible to have an operation to replace the aortic valve. She needed it soon.

This was not what Julia wanted to hear. She had left it late to have kids. After three months of excitement and expectation, she had become attached to her fetus. What if she never had another chance? She felt fine as long as she was doing nothing. Surely she could just do nothing until the baby was born. Simple logic. A price worth paying. But wrong. The cardiologist had no doubt. If nothing was done, both Julia and the baby would die long before it could be delivered. Even if it was delivered prematurely in twenty weeks' time. The options were few. No surgeon would operate on her aortic valve while she was pregnant. If she wanted, he would discuss her case at a multidisciplinary team meeting at the NHS hospital the following day. A group of cardiologists, surgeons, intensive-care doctors, and in Julia's case, obstetricians who would review the information in detail. Consider the options. Do the right thing.

But Julia was no wilting violet. "What about my opinion?" came the reply. "I want to keep my baby, not have people ganging up on me. What is my best chance of keeping the baby?" Not an easy question to answer. He thought for a minute and suggested referring her to a doctor in Oxford who specializes in heart problems during pregnancy.

The ethical principles pertaining to pregnancy are straightforward. The doctor's first responsibility is to the mother. It is acceptable to sacrifice a baby in utero to sustain the mother's health. It is not acceptable to put a mother at risk for the sake of an unborn child. A baby will normally survive if delivered after thirty weeks. Even twenty-eight weeks. Only rarely have dying mothers been kept alive with the sole objective of sustaining a fetus. The cardiologists at the district general hospital saw the echo images. They judged the valve to be far too tight for Julia to reach thirty weeks' gestation for a Caesarean section. The hormonal changes and the increase in blood volume were already life-threatening. She would not survive another sixteen weeks. They all agreed. Julia should be advised to have a termination of pregnancy within days. Then have the aortic valve replaced soon afterward. An abortion would turn a complex problem into a simple one. If you judge cardiac surgery to be simple.

The cardiologist phoned her at work that Thursday afternoon. He summarized the consensus from his colleagues. That "sorry" word again. But. He had arranged the appointment to see Dr. Oliver Ormerod in Oxford the following afternoon. On the NHS. He emphasized that there was no time to spare. And that she absolutely must not ride or exercise.

Getting to the appointment was a nightmare. Traffic was lined up on the highway to get into the hospital. More traffic lines to get into the parking lots. No parking spaces, no help. She was going to be late for the most important appointment of their two lives. She had the crushing chest pain again. Followed by crippling anxiety. Last Friday, she was an excited mother to be. Now she was filled with impending doom.

Oliver changed all that. No suit. No tie. Not serious. He reminded Julia of one of her childhood favorites: Popeye the sailor man. He was altogether different, he made her feel she was special in that consulting room. "You want to keep your baby? Let's see how we can help you with that." The chest tightness went. A wave of relaxation flowed through her body. Her hand involuntarily dropped down to the little bump. As if to say, "Don't worry. This doctor will look after us both."

What were the possibilities to keep Julia safe and the baby alive? Oliver agreed that the valve operation could not wait until the baby was viable at twenty-eight weeks' gestation. Therefore, the valve would have to be dealt with while trying to preserve the pregnancy. There were two potential ways forward. The first was a balloon dilatation, or valvuloplasty, of the critically narrowed valve orifice as a temporizing maneuver. The second was to proceed with open-heart surgery on the heart-lung machine. All previous opinion had been against the latter. Balloon dilatation, was done in the catheter laboratory under X-ray guidance, but the uterus could be shielded from the radiation. The balloon is inflated within the narrowed valve orifice to split and open the fused parts. If this would carry Julia through to thirty weeks, the valve could be replaced after the baby was delivered. She would then face safer heart surgery as a new mother.

One of my colleagues, now Professor Banning, was an expert with balloon valve interventions. Oliver needed more detailed echo pictures of the valve to show him. If he agreed, it would be done early the following week. What were the risks? The valve might split and leak badly, causing acute heart failure. A surgical team would need to stand by in the operating theaters. Alternatively, the valve might not open sufficiently to make a difference. Either way, there was a significant risk to the mother and baby. It was not straightforward. Oliver decided to admit her to the cardiology ward after the weekend. In the meantime, he would talk to the only surgeon he knew who had operated on patients in similar circumstances.

Oliver called me at home on that Friday evening. We talked about previous experience. The last pregnant patient we managed between us had an unusual murmur discovered at twenty-eight weeks. She was found to have a massive but benign tumor in the left atrium. A left atrial myxoma, like Anna's. We watched carefully for four weeks in the hospital, then delivered the baby by Caesarean section in a cardiac operating theater at thirty-two weeks. Three days later, I removed the tumor. Both did well. Before that, we had treated a young woman with an infected artificial-heart valve that was disintegrating and leaking badly. We took her to the operating theater at thirty-three weeks' gestation and performed the Caesarean section. Then I re-replaced the aortic valve at the same sitting. Mother and baby did well, though we had problems with bleeding from the uterus.

Then I reminded Oliver that I had replaced an aortic valve in a thirty-five-year-old with a twenty-week fetus in another hospital. The valve replacement was fine, and the baby had a detectable heart beat afterward. But in the middle of the night, the mother aborted and hemorrhaged profusely. We came close to losing the mother as well as the baby. Heart surgery in pregnancy is one of those rare procedures in which you can actually lose two patients. I had read and analyzed every published report about heart surgery during pregnancy. Then produced a detailed review. At the time, there were only 133 cases worldwide. Only nineteen were aortic valve replacements. No mothers had died, but seven of the babies were lost. Not reassuring. The problem is that surgeons prefer to report successes. There could be hundreds of unreported cases where the babies or even the mothers had died. Best kept quiet. But at least we had some statistics to share with Julia and her family.

Oliver asked what I thought about the balloon option. I said it was a good idea, but there were practical issues. Most congenitally deformed aortic valves don't have defined parts that would separate under balloon pressure—not like rheumatic mitral valves, where the technique was well established. It was a blind procedure. The valve might be destroyed. The aorta might split and bleed torrentially. We needed to ask Banning what he thought about the chances of success. If they decided to take the valvuloplasty route, I would do my best to provide backup. We left it there.

After the weekend, Julia was brought back into the hospital for more tests. News of the pregnancy conundrum spread fast. So there was a massive turnout at the congenital heart team meeting. This was the crack of dawn, Thursday morning. We were joined by pediatric cardiology colleagues from Southampton. Oliver presented the case with superb new pictures of her heart. The aortic valve orifice was a narrow slit. Instead of having three cusps, there appeared to be only one. What we call a monocusp valve. It looked like a rocky volcano. Almost 1 centimeter in depth, and rigid. The muscle below was ominously thick. It was remarkable that she had reached age forty in this state. Would the balloon make a difference? Unlikely. Was it safe? Unlikely. Then the bottom line. They had already made their decision. She should go directly for aortic valve replacement with a biological prosthetic valve—a valve that does not need anticoagulation that would endanger the pregnancy. This is what Julia wanted. It had been her decision. She disliked uncertainty. Not just feisty, but brave. No one in the meeting disagreed.

Would I do it? It had to be quick. The shortest possible time on the heart-lung machine. Although cardiopulmonary bypass is perfectly safe for the mother, it often proves the trigger for fetal death.

The uterus and placenta don't like it. The clear fluid that is used to fill the bypass machine dilutes the mother's blood. This dilutional effect drops the concentration of the pregnancy hormone progesterone. There is increased uterine irritability. When uterine contractions appear during cardiopulmonary bypass, that is an important predictor of fetal death. Next, the fetal heart rate decreases through decreased placental blood supply. Low oxygen levels in the baby's bloodstream can trigger a distress response. This raises blood pressure and puts pressure on the developing fetal heart. Often it fails to recover.

I explained how to manage cardiopulmonary bypass in the pregnant woman. We needed to use higher pressure and flow than normal. And avoid cooling so that the placental blood vessels wouldn't constrict. Expedited surgery was vital. The cardioplegia solution that would be needed to protect Julia's thickened heart muscle contained high levels of potassium. The baby's heart would be sensitive to elevated potassium. Too much maternal cardioplegia could stop it. So we should monitor the fetal heart rate and uterine contractions. If we detected contractions, we could infuse the pregnancy hormone progesterone to damp these down. Or increase the heart-lung machine flow if the fetal heart rate dropped. As long as everyone knew precisely what to expect, I felt we had a good chance of keeping the baby alive.

By now the mood had shifted away from terminating the pregnancy toward keeping the little family together. But we needed back-up. Should the baby die and spontaneously abort during the night, the gynecologists needed to be prepared. They might need to treat uterine bleeding in a patient who had just had heart surgery. The departments were in different buildings, but at least on the same campus. The following day was Friday. Not a good day to operate, with locum doctors and agency nurses working the weekend. I needed the best team I could muster. Julia was perfectly stable. We should do it on Monday morning. No fuss. Just another aortic valve replacement but with a careful plan and the right preparation.

What makes a quick surgeon? Not haste or rapid hand movements. In fact, the opposite. Being well organized. Not doing unnecessary things. Putting every stitch where it needs to be. Not having to repeat anything. Quick surgeons don't move fast. It is a matter of connection between brain and fingertips. You have to be born that way. No amount of training helps with this.

Now I needed to meet her. Oliver took me to Julia's room on the cardiology ward. She was alone. No family there in the morning. As promised, she was feisty and probing. But anxious about what I might say. Nervous that others had repeatedly argued for termination. Her first words were, "I want to keep the baby." I said, "I want to keep the baby, too." With this, we had a working relationship. I told her about the type of valve and that she wouldn't need anticoagulation. That was important for the later stages of pregnancy and delivery. But the valve would wear out. She would need another one in fifteen years' time. Maybe less. Julia wasn't thinking that far ahead. She just wanted this horrific intrusion removed from her ordered life. "Can I go home for the weekend?" she asked. To make some arrangements and let her employer know. "Okay but no riding, no exertion—of any kind! And not until we cross-match blood and the anesthetist comes in to see you." Oliver agreed. There was no point arguing with Julia. Monday's anesthetist was Elaine. I explained the delicate situation, and she came directly. While Elaine talked to Julia, I went to warn the perfusionists and give them some literature. Said what I wanted and emphasized that two lives were at risk this time.

When I next saw Julia at 7:00 a.m. on Monday, she was perfectly calm. She asked me to save the deformed valve. It belonged to her. She wanted to keep it. Her whole family was in the room. Husband, sister, and elderly parents. There for morale support. I said I would come back and talk to them later.

Now for the operation. The arterial and venous monitoring cannulas were put in using local anesthetic. I really didn't want to monitor the fetal heart rate. I had done all that before. It is a source of anxiety and distraction if the rate slows, and there is nothing we can do to change things when we are already taking the appropriate precautions. Elaine was being careful to keep the blood pressure and oxygen levels up during anesthetic induction. We had checked the fetal heart rate before taking Julie through into the operating theater. It was normal. One hundred and forty beats per minute. Twice that of the mother. The echo probe was pushed down the gullet and into Julia's stomach, ready to view the heart. We kept her covered with blankets until the last minute. To avoid cooling. Then off with everything. The little abdominal bump was there to remind the team to stay focused. Soon she had been painted with antiseptic and covered in blue drapes.

We worked our way down the layers: skin, fat, bone, marrow, and into the pericardium. Elaine gave the heparin in readiness for cardiopulmonary bypass. We inserted the cannulas through snares in the aorta and right atrium. Then on to cardiopulmonary bypass: we stopped ventilating the lungs, and the machine took over. Instead of cooling, we used the heat exchanger to keep her warm. And high pump flow to keep the uterus and placenta happy. With a clamp across the aorta, in went the heart-stopping cardioplegia fluid until the heart stopped dead. Not really dead, but flaccid and cold. Protected by stopping its metabolism.

I used a scalpel to slit open the aorta and expose the offending valve. It was not recognizable as a valve. Just as the echo predicted, it was a rock-solid volcano with a narrow slit. I cored it out in one piece with a different sharp-pointed blade. My gift to Julia, in a bottle of preserving fluid. Then I sewed in the new biological valve with twelve separate stitches. A valve carefully constructed from the pericardium of a cow. Suspended from a plastic frame with a sewing ring. Sewn onto where the old valve had been removed. A common, uncomplicated operation benefiting two patients. One present. One future. It was going well.

We sewed up the aorta and removed the clamp. Warm blood flooded into her coronary arteries. The heart was reanimated by lifeblood. First squirming in ventricular fibrillation. Then sudden spontaneous defibrillation. It lay perfectly still until I poked it. Then it contracted and ejected blood. After poking it again, normal heart rhythm began. The echo probe showed the artificial valve opening and closing, the way out of the left ventricle now wide open for the first time in decades. Thousands of small air bubbles dashed toward the needle. Routine and unexciting is precisely what we needed. I told Elaine to start ventilating the lungs, to check the blood gases and get ready to come off the machine. She rhythmically pumped air into the windpipe. The collapsed lungs filled with air and expanded. From flaccid and empty to inflated, pink, and proud. Surrounding the heart, same as always. Day after day. We stop life and start it again. Make things better. Take calculated risks.

A pulse wave returned to the arterial pressure trace. Now regular and strong. But I didn't look at the screen. I watched the heart itself. It was still pushing out residual air bubbles. They floated upward, straight into the right coronary artery. Coalescent air obstructed it. The right ventricle lost its blood supply and temporarily distended. No big deal. We increased pump flow and blood pressure to push the air through. The right ventricle contracted again. All is well. Now I wanted to get off the machine as soon as possible. I told the perfusionist to slowly ease off bypass. Let Julia's re-plumbed heart take over. We were on the machine for just forty-nine minutes. During that time, we maintained high flow rates and normal temperature. Did our best to look after the uterus and its precious cargo. I heard, "Off bypass." We removed the cannulas and reversed the heparin anticoagulant with protamine.

The cut surfaces were still bleeding. More than usual. My irritable bladder kicked in. It was best to let Mohammed finish off. Cauterize the bleeding sites. Put the drains and pacing wire in. Make sure she is safe. We were trying to avoid blood transfusion with its negative effects, but at the same time we must not allow oxygen delivery to be compromised. Too few red cells—not enough oxygen. Eventually we needed to give two units of donor blood, and fresh frozen plasma with its clotting factors. Then the sticky cells, called platelets, that plug the small holes. Within an hour, she was ready to transfer to the ICU. Bleeding under control.

The rest of the story: Elaine and Mohammed escorted her out of the operating theater complex. Elated that everything had gone according to plan. Yet after all the preparation, they were greeted by an inexperienced nurse. The ICU had been warned like everybody else. It wasn't the poor nurse's fault, but Elaine was irritated. What was the plan to look after the baby? When was the most likely time for the baby to die? What would we do if Julia had a torrential bleed down below? Blank faces. Wide-eyed nurses. Stupefied junior doctors. So get an experienced team together and get focused. I was oblivious to all this at the time, but Elaine was right. Experience matters a great deal in high-risk situations, and in this case two lives were at risk.

Julia's blood pressure was on the low side. Her blood vessels were more dilated than usual because we had kept her unusually warm on the bypass machine. The usual drugs we used to increase pressure would constrict the blood vessels to the uterus and placenta. We couldn't use them. Nor could we allow an average blood pressure at less than 70 mm Hg. The solution was in my written guideline. Everybody had it. Did anyone in the ICU read it? No point saying anything. Otherwise there would be a complaint. Bullying, offensive behavior, the usual NHS stuff. I asked Mohammed to stay with her. Oliver used an ultrasound machine to image the fetal heart. It was still beating away. Around 140 beats per minute. So far we had a viable fetus. And no uterine contractions. I told them to let her wake up and be taken off the breathing machine. Get rid of the sedative drugs. Then the blood pressure would rise spontaneously. I left to operate on the next patient, but I offered a parting shot—"You are looking after two people now. Not just the one you can see."

Julia woke up quickly and eventually had the tube removed from her windpipe. She described being awake with the tube down her windpipe as the worst part of the whole experience. I met Oliver at 7:00 a.m. the following morning to image the fetal heart. It was still bounding away at 140 beats per minute. Not just that, but the fetus was doing somersaults in the womb. Julia's heart was working well with the new valve. She had warm feet and a good volume of urine in the catheter bag. Ours is the only profession where piss makes us happy. But I was still uneasy. Her blood pressure was on the low side. No one knows enough about heart surgery in pregnancy to know if this mattered at this stage. We still didn't want to use drugs that would compromise the placental blood supply.

Julia's first question was "Is my baby still okay?" We reassured her that it seemed to be but looked forward to finding a strong heartbeat in another twenty-four hours. I felt we would be in the clear by then. Later that morning, we took the drain out of her chest. She was desperate to get back to a single room on the ward, but I wanted her blood pressure and oxygen levels monitored for another twenty-four hours. We moved her to a quiet isolation room normally used for septic patients. The next day, the fetus was still the same. Moving and with a normal heart rate. Julia was uncomfortable. The second postoperative day is the worst. Why not the first? Because the first day brings the euphoria of survival. The second just pain. For the baby's sake, we couldn't give her a heavy analgesic regime.

We operated on Monday. By Friday, Julia was bored, almost comfortable, and insisting on going home. We couldn't stop her. A concerned Oliver called her each day for the next week, then saw her regularly in the Outpatient Department. Fetal ultrasound scans showed normal growth and activity. Five months later, in January 2016, she delivered a nine-pound healthy baby boy. Her miracle child. Once destined to be an aborted fetus. We changed all that, Oliver and I. Welcome to the world, Samson. Strong man! An appropriate name under the circumstances.

sixteen Your Life in
Their Hands

Have a heart that never hardens, and a temper
that never tires, and a touch that never hurts.

—Charles Dickens

I‍T WAS 2004. ALMOST FIFTY YEARS SINCE A TELEVISION PRO-
gram had planted the seed in my brain and shaped my destiny.
The BBC called my office and spoke with secretary Dee. She was
excited when I returned between cases. Would I consider doing a
program for them? A full hour of prime-time television all about me.
They were looking for a brain surgeon, a transplant surgeon, and
a heart surgeon for three separate episodes. I was stunned when I
heard the name of the series: *Your Life in Their Hands*.

The distinguished producer and his assistant came to Oxford to
talk through the implications. They explained that the filming could
be intrusive for a while. They would spend six months with me. At
the hospital and at home. Meeting the patients. Interacting with
my family. So the viewers could appreciate how it felt to be a heart

surgeon. Life at the sharp end. In my case, very sharp. They wanted me to implant a Jarvik 2000 for the cameras. Would I please find them an appropriate heart-failure patient to follow? Before, during, and after the operation. Of course, they would feature other cases. They would like a baby case, and other dramatic high-risk stuff. Cutting edge, inspirational surgery in real time. They would do the filming and decide which material to use. They had done their background research. They knew that I regularly operated live for surgical audiences. That I was flamboyant and a confident performer. Not easily intimidated. If I agreed to do it, they would make the arrangements with the hospital. At the time, we had a chief executive who talked to us. A likeable guy who periodically emerged from the Ivory Tower to visit the worker bees. I had no doubt that he would agree. Now I just had to let my family know that a film crew would be coming home with me after work. And meeting me in the mornings. And interviewing them. How was it to live with a heart surgeon? Good question!

It became normal to have a film crew on my shoulder. Many operations were recorded. Premature babies with holes in the heart. Young adults needing massive surgery for aortic aneurysms in the inherited condition called Marfan's syndrome. A middle-aged woman needing her fifth aortic valve replacement, a difficult procedure that eventually took twenty-four hours. Things went dramatically wrong on-camera, but she survived. Of course they used that material. They filmed me jogging with Mark and watching Gemma play golf for Cambridge University. But after months of this, there was still no suitable candidate for the Jarvik 2000. Eventually, I called Philip Poole-Wilson at the Royal Brompton Hospital. It took him less than a week to locate the ideal patient—a delightful fifty-eight-year-old Scotsman who had already been turned down for transplantation in Glasgow. Jim Braid was very much in the mold of Peter Houghton. He was dying but desperately wanted to survive long enough to see his daughter graduate from college and get married one day. As the clock ticked on relentlessly, it was becoming clear that he wouldn't make it.

It had been a long time since Jim's transplant assessment. We needed up-to-date information. Philip brought him down from Scotland and admitted him to the Brompton. He needed repeat right and left heart catheterization, detailed echocardiography, and lots of blood tests. I was mindful of the fact that we were still paying for all of this out of charitable funds. The NHS wouldn't pay. It had written him off like Peter and the others. I was his only chance. Glasgow was correct about him being unsuitable for a heart transplant. The blood pressure in his lungs was too high. Yet Jim's own right ventricle was used to it. It was his left ventricle that was deteriorating. He had the same problem as Peter. Dilated cardiomyopathy. Neither were the kidneys working well enough to tolerate the immunosuppressive drugs that a heart transplant would need. A left ventricular assist device would take over from his flabby, failing heart. Not only that—it might help to rejuvenate it. Possibly. The echo showed it certainly couldn't afford to get any worse. It was now or never. We couldn't risk letting him go home to Scotland.

I took the excited BBC team down to Fulham Road to meet Jim and his wife, Mary. Peter Houghton came down from Birmingham. He was in great form, still raising money so that others could have pumps. It was now four years since his implant, and that was close to surpassing the world record for survival with any type of artificial heart. Peter was pleased to counsel Jim and Mary. He did this professionally and liked to be regarded as part of the team. They were justifiably nervous but eager to proceed, suitably impressed with the technology. Moreover, Jim was a great character. Perfect for television. He could barely speak, and his nose and lips were blue. He shuffled down the corridors, head bowed, panting for breath. But he would joke for the camera. He said, "It's great to be down in London with these Ferrari mechanics. Not like the Ford Escort boys up north." That resonated with me. It was good to be back at the

Brompton. At Oxford, we had already lost most of the original intensive-care team. They had moved on. I asked Philip if we could do the implant there, in London. That pleased him enormously. First, I needed to engage with the senior surgeon, Professor John Pepper. He was happy to help out, so we planned the operation for the following week. Rob Jarvik agreed to fly the pump across from New York at short notice. My Oxford colleague Andrew Freeland would come to help with the skull pedestal. Now we had the patient, the pump, and a top team. The producer's dream. All we needed was a successful implant with those cameras rolling. Jim must survive. Yet he wasn't fit for an anesthetic. The Brompton anesthetists emphasized that. Nevertheless, the hospital remained enthusiastic and supportive. We didn't have to fight the management to do it. That hospital had never implanted a left ventricular assist device before and would have been disappointed if we didn't go ahead.

Five thirty in the morning. Dark and cold. The film crew picked me up by taxi, and we headed into Oxford to find Andrew. He was wandering down Woodstock Road, carrying instruments to screw the plug into Jim's skull. We drove down the M40, doing an interview in the car. "How did I feel about operating at a different hospital?" "Excited." I had operated everywhere from Tehran to Toronto. An operating theater is an operating theater and I had a good team. As Baldrick would say in Blackadder, "We have a cunning plan!" "How did I feel about the fact that he could easily die? Was I nervous?" "Absolutely not. Jim would be dead in days if we didn't try. No one else was going to help." "Did I think that the NHS should pay for these pumps?" I answered that with a question of my own. "Should a First World health care system use modern technology to prolong life? Or should it let young heart-failure patients die miserably? As in the Third World?" The BBC liked that answer but didn't broadcast it in the program. Too controversial.

We arrived at the Brompton at 7:00 a.m. I took Andrew and the crew directly to the deserted canteen. Little had changed since my day. They still did a good breakfast. I helped myself to the healthy option. Sausage, bacon, black pudding, fried egg, and fried bread. Andrew followed suit. As we sat together, the cameras started rolling. It was what the producer was waiting for. Heart doctor eats huge pile of fried food. Wall-to-wall cholesterol. I said, "This is great. I never get this at home." Andrew responded, "What would your wife say about that?" My answer, "Don't care!" This encounter turned out to be what everyone remembered about the program. When my brain surgeon friend Henry Marsh did his episode, they filmed him cycling to work through the streets of London. Without a crash helmet! When asked, he simply stated "Never wear one. It wouldn't save me!" The BBC wanted characters. They got characters.

John Pepper came down to meet us. Under the circumstances we were a very relaxed group. Perhaps not what you might expect, but good for Jim. Stressed surgeons do not function well. Numerous studies show that. Stress impairs judgment and makes the hands shake. Stress is killing my profession. We went to the ward to see Jim and Mary before they brought him down. Jim was excited. Mary was petrified. Was this her last good-bye? The end of their journey together? Would it be the high road or the low road back to Scotland? I did what I always do. Reassured them that everything would be fine. Not that I knew that. I just wanted them to go into the operation with confidence. With the cameras rolling, we were all in this together.

There was an air of busy excitement in the operating theater. Nurses setting up trays of glistening instruments. Perfusionists assembling their heart-lung machine. A technician jealously guarding the artificial heart. Only to be revealed at the crucial time. But no Lord Brock's boots this time. I was my own man.

Now uncovered, poor Jim was obviously emaciated from the heart failure. The left side of his head was shaved and ready for the skull pedestal and power line. He was about to become battery-powered. John inserted the pipes for the cardiopulmonary bypass machine into the main artery and vein of Jim's left leg. He began with needle and guidewire, then small stab wounds. This was more sophisticated equipment than mine. With my equipment, we still needed to make surgical incisions to expose the vessels. I was learning something. Once Jim's chest was prepared with iodine and draped with adhesive film, Andrew exposed the surface of the skull while I sliced open the ribs. The camera panned from one site to the other. About a liter of fluid poured out of Jim's chest. Heart-failure juice. Then I could see the hugely dilated left ventricle through the pericardial sac. There was fluid in there, too. I started to tunnel the pump's electric drive line out through the apex of the chest and into the neck. Avoiding the perilous blood vessels and nerves to the left arm. Once through the neck, I delivered the miniature plug on the end to Andrew. He would pass this through the middle of the titanium skull pedestal, then screw the titanium onto the skull behind the ear. Rigid fixation. So that the external power line could be plugged in securely. Fascinating on film, but we still hadn't reached the tricky bit.

As I opened the pericardium, clear fluid spilled out. The pale, distended left ventricle twitched. You couldn't dignify it with the word *contraction*. I urged the cameraman to focus in on it. I was about to sew on the pump's restraining cuff. Each time the needle pierced the muscle, the heart quivered in response and threatened to fibrillate. This was irritating because I was trying to do the implant without starting the heart-lung machine. This would reduce the risk of bleeding at the end of the operation. But Jim was too unstable. Before the cuff was secure, the heart did fibrillate. No blood pressure, but no problem. We started the bypass machine and emptied the heart.

Now came the exciting sequence for the film. Carving the hole in the apex of the heart to insert the Jarvik 2000. First I made the cruciate scalpel incision where blood always spurts out. Next, I cored out a circle of muscle with a cork bore device, causing blood to pour into the pericardium. Then insertion of the titanium pump into the heart, which stops the bleeding. With a professor of surgery assisting me, this all went smoothly. Andrew connected the external power cable to the skull pedestal, and we switched Jim on. Slowly at first, until blood expelled the air from the Dacron graft. As usual, air comes fizzing and frothing out of the needle. Red bubbles on the white tube. Visually satisfying. I instructed the perfusionist to cut back on flow. To fill the heart before turning up the Jarvik 2000 impeller speed. The last air bubbles spluttered out from the highest part of the ventricle. Apex uppermost. Simple physics and done without thinking. Lots of chemistry was going on at the same time. Optimizing the potassium level. Neutralizing the lactic acid with sodium bicarbonate. Then biology. Electrical defibrillation of the quivering muscle to provide a stable heart rhythm. My three school examination subjects were not wasted.

For many viewers, it was the engineering that proved exciting. An electric plug in the head. A turbine in the heart. Spinning at 12,000 rpm without damaging the blood cells. No pulse. I maintained a continuous commentary for the television while throwing out instructions to the anesthetist and perfusionists. "Start ventilating the lungs. Reduce your flow. Turn up the Jarvik." Detailed coordination by a guy who couldn't lift a car hood or use a computer. No one could quite believe how well this had gone.

I regularly grapple with the tension between altruism and self-interest in high-risk cases, but in this instance it was both. Naively, I thought that if the public could see Jim's miraculous recovery, there would be pressure to treat patients on the NHS. We couldn't sustain a charitably funded program any longer. This was secondhand-shop health care. Poole-Wilson had this in mind, too. We wanted to do a proper clinical trial by randomly allocating dying heart-failure patients to a ventricular assist device or continued medical treatment. We knew what the outcome would be. Symptom-free extended life, versus inexorable deterioration and death. We didn't consider that fair to those who didn't get a pump, but the devices would never be approved for NHS use without a trial.

Only the British Heart Foundation had enough money to support this endeavor. The organization turned us down. At the time it couldn't be done in America, where people were waiting to see the long-term outcome of pulseless patients before agreeing to it. All eyes were on us.

Jim separated easily from the bypass machine. This was the most taxing part for the Brompton anesthetists. It was the first time they had managed a patient with continuous blood flow. An average "flat-line" blood pressure of 80 mm Hg was optimum. For any other heart patient, this would be regarded as unreasonably low. Vasoconstrictor drugs would normally be used to raise it beyond 100 mg Hg, but Jim needed a counterintuitive approach. We gave him vasodilator drugs to reduce blood pressure. We had learned all this through trial and error. It worked in the laboratory. It should be fine on the wards. Albeit a source of fascination for the Brompton team and the film crew.

Andrew closed the scalp and neck incisions, then took off for Oxford. He had a busy clinic that afternoon. Snotty noses and wax-filled ears. Not artificial hearts. John removed the pipes from the groin. I inserted the chest drains and started to close the chest wound. Meticulously cauterizing all the bleeding points. The scalp was still oozing. I put a couple of extra stitches to the skin and cleaned blood from the skull pedestal. Today, cosmetics mattered. We needed clean white dressings and empty drains. Every spot of blood cleaned away. Nostalgically, I remembered my first heart operation in this very same operating theater. Wearing Lord Brock's boots. When I pushed the saw through the poor lady's sternum and into the heart. Mattias Paneth strolling through the theater doors in his pin-striped suit. Exclaiming, "Westaby, what have you done this time?" Now it was me in charge.

The cameras kept rolling as Jim was wheeled off to the ICU. I glanced back into that operating theater for the last time. There were pools of blood under the table. Glistening bright red under the lights.

And a puddle of urine where the catheter bag had leaked. The perfusionists were folding their redundant tubes into a yellow plastic container. Bloodied green drapes were being stuffed into clear plastic bags. The nurses in their theater blues were disposing of their bloodied instruments and used swabs. All colors of the rainbow. An artist's dream. A historic day. The backstreet kid from Scunthorpe had implanted an artificial heart at the Brompton. For the television program that took him there in the first place. Thirty years before.

Once Jim was safely connected to the ventilator and monitors, we went to find Mary and her daughter. There was no escape from the cameras. Drama they were after, and drama they were determined to find. We took the family to see Jim. The surroundings in critical care are always intimidating, this time particularly so with Jim's scalp shaved and a black power cable dangling from his head. Life dependent on a battery. We explained everything to them, but they already knew most of it from Peter Houghton. Peter was on his way to the hospital. But they couldn't see the electric plug under his hair. It was rather more alarming to confront it head on. I handed Jim's daughter a stethoscope and placed the listening end over his heart. A look of surprise lit up her face. She could hear the continuous whine of the spinning impeller that would keep her dad alive. I pointed to the cardiac output monitor. It was pumping 4 liters of blood per minute. Consuming 7 watts of power via the controller and battery. I could turn Jim's blood flow up or down with one single knob. The producer loved it. This was much more exciting than brain surgery. Drilling small holes in the head and sucking out bits of tumor! That needs a different personality type altogether.

Jim stayed incredibly, boringly stable. He didn't bleed, whereas Peter and others lost gallons. John, Philip, and I wistfully discussed other potential patients. Where could we get the money? I could raise enough for a few more pumps but not a full-scale trial. The discussions ended up where they needed to. In the pub. Cameras and all. When I wandered back to the ICU, Peter Houghton was with the family. Beaming like a Cheshire cat. It was important for him to have what he called "cyborg companions." Battery-driven people making a new life for themselves. Frankenstein's monsters with a metal bolt sticking out of their skull. For me, this was a happy scene. One day all life would be this way. With that curious note of fantasy, I decided to go home to Woodstock. The longer I stayed at the Brompton, the more I wished I worked there. It was a famous old hospital wanting to do new things. Not seeking reasons not to do them.

I operated in Oxford the next day, then headed back to London. Jim had been taken off the ventilator. The tube was out of his windpipe, and he was chatting to Mary. He looked completely different. Animated and radiating joy. His nose and ears were pink, not blue. Back in the land of the living. Now the pump was pushing out 5 liters of blood per minute. No pulse on the arterial pressure trace. And there was a liter of urine in the bag, which meant the kidneys were happy. By now the camera team was in the pub. I asked the intensive-care doctor whether he had prescribed warfarin yet. It was all done. There was nothing for me to add. This dead-end heart failure patient was recovering rapidly. No need for immunosuppression or the other poisons that a heart-transplant patient needs. What's more, Jim's own right ventricle was coping well with the extra blood flow. I went back to Woodstock with a sense of deep satisfaction.

I saw Jim several times before he returned to Scotland. Philip greatly reduced his heart-failure drugs, in particular the water tablets that make every patient's life difficult. The family had no problem getting used to the pump, changing the batteries regularly and plugging him into the electric supply overnight. His ankles slimmed down. He was no longer breathless. Jim could lie flat for the first time in months. Weeks later, he was there when his daughter graduated from her university. With a glass of champagne in his hand. Then the BBC filmed him walking along a Scottish beach with Mary at sunset. A happy man breathing easily, reflecting on his journey.

They used that poignant scene to close the program. The *Your Life in Their Hands* series won a prestigious award for Best Television Documentary. I was proud to play my part in that. It was a high point in my career.

Only rarely did Jim return to the Brompton for a checkup. The local hospital and his GP became familiar with the technology and were happy to look after him. Then sad news from Scotland. It was shortly before Christmas. Jim had gone to visit a friend without taking a spare battery. He was enjoying life, and his mind was on other things. The "low power" alarm went off on the controller. This meant that he had twenty minutes to change the battery before the power went off altogether. Jim didn't make it home. His own heart had not recovered sufficiently to see him through. When the battery expired, Jim died, too. His lungs filled with fluid. It was desperately sad after three years of good-quality extra life. For me, this catastrophe illustrated just how effective these devices can be. It was another tragic loss. This was the last permanent heart pump I implanted.

In the prevailing economic climate in the NHS, I could no longer rely on charity. It became a serious risk to my own family. That meant the end of our pioneering efforts for patients but the beginning of my quest to develop affordable artificial-heart technology in the laboratory. Now I was in the unenviable position of having to sit back and watch patients die—people I once could have saved. Misery. It takes some getting used to.

Time passes. Before I knew it, it was 2016. By now I'd had a lifetime in cardiac surgery. How much longer did I want to spend doing this? The trouble was that I remained good at it. I was still a compulsive operator who would take on the difficult stuff, vastly experienced in the way new surgeons could never be. Did I owe it to the patients to stay? Or to my family to quit? Move to an easier job. My brain and retirement were not compatible.

Yet my body was telling me to stop. My right hand was deformed. The fascia in my palm was contracting. It was turning into a claw hand, known as Dupuytren's contracture. Frozen by scar tissue where the scrub nurse slapped the metal instruments into my palm. Now I couldn't even shake hands properly. It was deformed into the position I used to hold the scissors, the needle holder, the sternal saw. A true occupational adaptation—but one that ultimately forced a decision. Then, as for many aging surgeons, bending over an operation table for hours on end eventually took a toll on my spine. As I used to instruct my residents, "Please take over—my back's bad and the front's not so good, either." Yet no physical ailment was as debilitating as hospital bureaucracy. Not being able to operate. No beds, not enough nurses, junior doctors on strike. Having to endure "Statutory and Mandatory" training that requires doctors to sit in a classroom while a paramedic teaches them how to resuscitate. Or having to take a quiz on how to prescribe insulin or cancer drugs. Things that I never even have to do. Or writing my personal development plan at the age of sixty-eight. All of it time wasted, when I should be up to my elbows in someone's chest—doing some good. After all, I am a glorified plumber. Do plumbers have to report annually on their personal development plan? Or plumb all night? Or attend plumbing conferences to collect their "Continuing Plumbing Education Points"? Check off boxes on a computer screen? Absolutely not. They make more money than NHS surgeons and retire at sixty. Does no one appreciate that irreplaceable senior medical staff are heading for the exit in droves? Oxford's only specialist heart-failure cardiologist left to train as a lawyer. Our world-class children's interventional cardiologist left for America. Archer and Forfar were leaving. Ormerod was close to that decision.

The fire alarm went off in the operating theaters recently. Right in the middle of a valve operation. The patient was still on the bypass machine. The heart cold and flaccid. The prosthetic valve half sewn in. An administrator poked her head around the door to say, "The fire alarm has gone off. We don't think there is a fire but we have to evacuate." I just said, "Right, then, I'm off." The look on her face was priceless. I followed up with, "You rush off, then. Save yourself but please leave us a bucket. We'll piss in it and put the fire out!" Hilarious laughter from the theater staff as Rome burns. "Lions led by donkeys," as they put it in World War I.

But it wasn't funny. One can only tolerate so much. My whole profession had lost direction.

Epilogue

Don't cry because it's over. Smile because it happened.

—Theodor Seuss Geisel

After I qualified in medicine in 1972, the old Charing Cross Hospital closed and relocated. When the last patient left the famous landmark on the Strand, many of us students walked around the empty shell to reminisce about our training. I went back to that rickety old elevator and up into the eaves. For one last time, I opened the green door into the Ether Dome. The electric lights still worked, but the dusty, antiquated equipment had gone. I walked tentatively to gaze over into the operating theater. As I had six years before, in 1966. Sure enough, that last spot of Beth's blood was there on top of the operating light. Black, ingrained, and inaccessible. They never did succeed in washing her away.

Beth continued to visit me in the dead of night. Particularly during bad times—of which there were many. The baby was now in her arms. Behind it the brutal metal retractor embedded in her frail chest. The dead heart empty and still. She would walk toward me, pallid and with piercing eyes. Beth wanted me to be a cardiac surgeon, and I didn't disappoint her. I was good at it. Yet despite my best efforts, some patients took the fast track to Heaven. How many, I really don't know. Like a bomber pilot, I didn't dwell on death. More than 300, less than 400, I guess. But Beth was my only ghost.

June 2016. An astonishing fifty years after I tentatively passed through the doors of the dissecting room as a nervous young student. To start cutting on a wizened, greasy, and embalmed human body. Now I was standing at a podium in the Royal College of Surgeons. Holding court at a meeting for heart surgeons in training. The organizers have paraded me out as a role model. Heart surgeon for thirty-five years without being sued or suspended. An increasingly rare species. My talk was about the illustrious history of the heart-lung machine and circulatory-support technology. Much about my colleagues in the United States. Celebrating the great men and daring deeds that I grew up with. Not to mention those I performed myself.

As the next lecture was beginning, I attempted to leave unnoticed. There was a flurry of activity behind. The scramble of eager young men who wanted their picture taken with me. I was flattered. We posed in front of the marble statue of John Hunter in the entrance hall. Legendary surgeon, anatomist, body snatcher. I always felt uneasy there. It was the spot where I learned that I had failed my exams. On more than one occasion. When my name wasn't read out. When many of us walked away in shame. Even my eventual triumph was painful. I took the oral examinations with a badly fractured jaw that kept me quiet. On a grim winter's afternoon in Cambridge, a misjudged rugby tackle had landed me in the Addenbrookes Accident Department, covered in mud. Still in my shorts, I was waiting to see the orthodontic surgeon when an ambulance brought in a young motorcycle-accident victim. He was bleeding to death into his left chest, and there was no time to call the chest surgeons from Papworth Hospital. The Emergency Department doctor and the nursing sister both knew I had worked there. They asked me to intervene before it was too late. So I opened him just as I was, wearing my rugby kit with muddy knees. Spitting out my own blood into the scrub sink. This bizarre story spread swiftly, and there were Cambridge surgeons at the examinations. Maybe it helped. Ultimate success didn't dim those memories. I detested the cardboard elitism. Examiners dressed in bright-red gowns sweeping around the pillars. Flash Gordon outfits, I used to call them. Now it had become an institution that tacitly supported the "name-and-shame" culture that endorsed the public release of named surgeons' death rates. That tipped its hat to the politicians who ruled health care in preference to defending its members.

How things had changed since my day. Despite the hardships, when you made it into heart surgery, you felt ten feet tall. Proud, bullish, like fighting cocks. You had reached the top. People respected you. These trainees were downtrodden. Defensive. Uncertain of themselves. So the mood in the college was somber. Out in the hall after my lecture, one earnest young resident of Middle Eastern origin wanted to talk. His hospital was under investigation for borderline results. His mentors, whom he respected, were being chastised in the newspapers. He wondered whether he should continue. Was it worth the struggle? Or should he give up and go home to his family? I told him that I had once operated on a sick, blue baby in Iran. The child of a politician back in the days after the revolution. At the time, I was worried about my own safety if the child did not survive. But I stuck my neck out because the patient had no other option. So I gave this young man my first piece of advice, "We are here for the patients, not for ourselves. We may suffer for that, but we will rarely regret it."

We left the gloom of that historic building and walked down to the Strand in the sun. I asked the young man why he had chosen heart surgery in the first place. He told me his sister had died from a congenital heart defect. He wanted to operate on children, but this al-ready seemed a "bridge too far." As we passed the Savoy, I recounted my own story. About losing my grandfather to heart failure and wanting to find a solution. If a backstreet kid from Scunthorpe could do it, so could he. Then I told him about Winston Churchill, whom I often talked with in Bladon churchyard. How in the dark days and during his "black dog" hours he never gave up. And how I didn't give up after the debacle of my own first heart operation. My second piece of advice: "Follow your star. Do it for your sister."

We diverted from the Strand past the Rules restaurant in Covent Garden. As an impecunious student, I would seek to impress potential girlfriends there. Then starve for the rest of the month. I told him not to be afraid to take risks. Sometimes they pay off handsomely. We walked for another hundred yards, and there was the entrance portal of the old Charing Cross Hospital. Now a police station. My glorious medical school turned into office buildings. I described to him the Ether Dome and the operation that haunted me. A catastrophe that could have changed my life. But it didn't. It made me more determined. To press on against the odds. So perhaps one more thought. The past is the past. Put it behind you. It is tomorrow that matters.

The young man was grateful. Taking the time to talk made a difference to him. Perhaps he felt as I did in America. When Dr. Kirklin told me to take the difficult route and operate on children. Or when Dr. Cooley showed me that first artificial heart. As the young man turned to go back to the conference, he tried to shake my hand. From his quizzical look, I could tell he was surprised at how badly it was deformed. Forty years of metal instruments being smacked into my palm. Until recently, it hadn't interfered with my operating. I had been advised to have surgery long before but typically had ignored it. Concerned that it would end my surgical career. Now it had gone too far. I could no longer grasp the instruments without dropping some of them. I couldn't shake hands without people thinking I was a member of some secret society. So I asked myself something. Sure, I had a glittering career, but did I ever have a life?

At that point, I conceded that my operating days were over. I would never get back to complex surgery. Instead I would focus on a new stem-cell project and the development of our own British ventricular assist device. Plenty to engage with, but different. It was then that I was made a professor at the Royal Brompton. To do research with the potential to change millions of lives. Just a few weeks later, I quietly disappeared from my hospital in Oxford and had that battered right hand operated on by a plastic surgeon. Normally, my colleagues would have done it using a regional nerve block with me awake. But they didn't want the interference.

I was pleased to be asleep. I didn't enjoy being on the other side of the fence. For me, it wasn't just an operation. It was the end of an era.

Acknowledgments

MY MENTOR IN THE UNITED STATES WAS THE GREAT Dr. John Kirklin, who launched open heart surgery with the heart–lung machine. Toward the end of his distinguished career he wrote:

> After many years of cardiac surgery, with many tests and challenges, and after many deaths that could not then be prevented, we tend gradually to become a little weary and, in some sense, infinitely sad because of life's inevitabilities.

I wrote this book because I've reached that same point in a career spanning the rise and fall of the NHS. Hence my acknowledgments are as emotionally charged as the rest of the text.

Heart surgery has been, in turn, a difficult road and a lonely destination. In the 1970s and 1980s, we really did work constantly. In the States it was 5:00 a.m. ward rounds, call the boss at 6:00 a.m., operate all day, go to the laboratory in the evenings, capped by nighttime vigils beside the intensive care bed. It was not so different at the Brompton or Hammersmith hospitals in London.

The pioneering early days were highly competitive, and junior heart surgeons were the thrusting young blades of the medical world. I was lucky. I succeeded because early in my training I learned from the great men: Roy Calne, John Kirklin, Denton Cooley, Donald Ross, Bud Frazier, and many more. I understood what was necessary to move the specialty forward. For me it took relentless effort and lateral thinking, then sheer guts to go with the blood.

This ruined any aspiration toward a normal family life. We were not normal people. Most rational young men would be paralyzed by fear at the thought of carving open someone's chest, then stopping, opening, and repairing the heart within. But I did this day after day. We were fueled with testosterone, driven by adrenaline. Few of us stayed married in our youth, and many of us subsequently harbored deep regrets.

I was always sorry for the distress caused to my first wife, Jane, and eternally grateful for my talented daughter, Gemma, now a Cambridge-educated human resources lawyer. While I spent many hours striving to save other people's children, I never spent enough time with my own. This book goes some way to explaining why I was so preoccupied. It also gives me the opportunity to emphasize that nothing ever mattered more to me than them—and the rest of my precious family. My only sibling, David, attended the same grammar school in Scunthorpe but did go to Cambridge. He read medicine at Christ's College, then followed me to Charing Cross and became an eminent gastroenterologist in London.

Inevitably, I met my soulmate over an open chest in the Accident Department, blood everywhere, drowning in sheer desperation. Sarah was the kindest accident and emergency sister I ever met. The daughter of a Battle of Britain Spitfire pilot, she was never flustered; nothing was too much effort. The young patient died, and when I couldn't face telling the family, she dealt with it. She did the same for others, time and time again. A free spirit from Africa, she made no distinction between tramps and politicians—they were all valued people to be treated with respect. I ruined her relationship and she suffered considerably for it. But she went on to give me unquestioning and unfailing love and support for the past thirty-five years, particularly through those difficult times. Mark came along ten years after Gemma, a sportsman and adventurer who took himself off to South Africa to train as a game ranger.

It was a struggle to build the Oxford program. The hard work was done by a handful of dedicated personnel who took the cardiac center from fewer than one hundred operations a year in 1986 to more than 1,600 in 2000. Our productivity was allied to innovation, and the team was replete with skilled surgeons and cardiologists, supportive anesthetists and perfusionists, and superb nurses—too many to name, but I'm grateful to all of them.

We could never have started the pediatric and artificial-heart programs without the support of one visionary hospital chief executive, Nigel Crisp, who went on to run the whole NHS and now deservedly sits in the House of Lords. Much of the artificial-heart work was undertaken with charitable funding. In that context, certain individuals and organizations were very generous. These include Heart Research UK; Sir Kirby Laing; Jim Marshall of Marshall Amplifiers (to whom I was introduced by my patient, the entertainer Frankie Vaughan); Christos Lazari; and the TI Group, courtesy of Sir Christopher Lewinton and David Lillycrop. I would also like to pay tribute to Professor Philip Poole-Wilson, past president at the European Society of Cardiology, who helped us greatly with the Jarvik 2000 Heart Program. Philip sadly passed away suddenly on his way to work at the Royal Brompton Hospital.

Eventually, when I was the only remaining pediatric surgeon, we lost children's heart surgery. Then I had to move the artificial-heart research away from Oxford.

I'm grateful to my friend Professor Marc Clement, head of both the Institute of Life Sciences and the Business School at the

University of Swansea for providing us with a laboratory and an engineering team. We met serendipitously through my famous artificial-heart patient Peter Houghton, who, with Nicki King, worked tirelessly to raise charitable research funding. Under the corporate banner Calon Cardio-Technology, we now have an implantable British ventricular assist device to compete with the American pumps, all of which cost the same as a Ferrari! Stuart McConchie, past chief executive of the HeartWare Company and Jarvik Heart, came to help us with that.

The Welsh connection put me in contact with the Nobel Prize–winning professor Sir Martin Evans of Cardiff University, who first isolated fetal stem cells. With his colleague Ajan Reginald and the company Celixir, he has worked on a heart-specific cell for regenerative medicine. With pumps and cells we aim to create a definitive alternative to heart transplantation.

Despite a degree in biochemistry and a PhD in the bioengineering of mechanical hearts, I'm a computer-illiterate technophobe who is unable to perform the simplest repair on a car. So I've relied on good old-fashioned secretaries. For the past ten years, Sue Francis has kept me afloat. We'd both be in the office before 6:30 a.m. Our Portakabin window looked directly onto the noisy twisted pipes of an air-conditioning plant, like an apocalyptic scene from Banksy's Dismaland. In summer, flying ants ate through the window frames, then in the winter the cold rain seeped through the holes. I spent long, restless nights there, scrunched up on a small sofa, afraid to go home in case my patient deteriorated. Besides my patients, world-famous people visited that office—Christiaan Barnard, Denton Cooley, Robert Jarvik, even David Cameron, our past prime minister. All were bewildered by the modesty of an NHS heart surgeon's headquarters. But between us, Sue and I achieved great things; she took home and typed hundreds of publications, not to mention this book.

In that context I'd like to thank John Harrison, who published some of my surgical textbooks. John encouraged me to write for the public and introduced me to my agent, Julian Alexander, who made this book happen. It was also a pleasure to work with the expertise of TJ Keller, Carrie Napolitano, Shena Redmond, and the rest of the team at Basic Books. I would also like to thank my medical artist, colleague, and friend, Dee McLean, for her superb illustrations.

So what happened to heart surgery in the United Kingdom? After multiple hospital scandals, the NHS in England decided to publish the death rates of individual surgeons. Now no one wants to be a heart surgeon. And who would, with the long, taxing operations, the anxious relatives, and the nights and weekends on call? It's a system entrenched in nonsensical bureaucracy, with the reward of public exposure for a run of bad luck. Already 60 percent of the children's heart surgeons in the United Kingdom are overseas graduates.

Ultimately, the stars of this book are my patients, but I fear that few of the dramatic cases would now reach an operating theater in the United Kingdom. In the final analysis, a profession that dwells upon death is unlikely to prosper, undertakers and the military apart. As Dr. Kirklin emphasized, death in cardiac surgery is inevitable. When surgeons remain focused on helping as many patients as their ability will allow, some patients will die. But we should no longer accept substandard facilities, teams, or equipment. Otherwise, patients will die needlessly. The comedian Hugh Dennis is not noted for his empathy. On the satirical BBC program *Mock the Week*, he offered an alternative ode to Dr. Kirklin's thoughtful statement:

> Roses are red,
> And Violets are blue.
> Sorry you're dead,
> What can I do?

The answer? Bury the blame-and-shame culture and give us the tools to do the job!

Glossary

AB-180 ventricular assist device: a centrifugal blood pump that was originally implanted into the chest. Now known as the Tandem Heart, an external temporary blood pump used in cardiogenic shock.

acute heart failure: the left ventricle fails rapidly and cannot sustain sufficient blood flow to the body. The lungs then fill with fluid. Usually caused by myocardial infarction or viral myocarditis and has a high mortality rate. See also *shock*.

angina: crushing pain in the chest, neck, and left arm due to limitation of blood flow to heart muscle in coronary artery disease. Typically comes on during exercise. If it comes on at rest, it may warn of a heart attack.

angiogram: cardiological investigation in which a long catheter is passed through the blood vessels into the heart. This allows blood pressure to be measured in the cardiac chambers and dye to be injected to visualize the coronary arteries or aorta.

aorta: large, thick-walled artery that leaves the left ventricle, then branches to supply the whole body. The first small branches are the coronary arteries, which supply blood to the heart itself.

aortic stenosis: narrowing of the aortic valve at the outlet of the left ventricle, restricting blood flow around the body. Can be caused by a congenital anomaly or degeneration in old age.

arteries: the blood vessels that convey blood to the organs and muscles of the body.

blood pressure: pressure within the large arteries. Normally measured by a cuff and stethoscope or a cannula inserted into an artery. Normal blood pressure is around 120/80mm Hg. The higher figure is when the left ventricle contracts; the lower, when it relaxes.

bridge to recovery: the process whereby a ventricular assist device is used to sustain the circulation and rest an acutely failing heart pending recovery from a reversible condition. If the heart does not recover, a limited-duration pump can be replaced by a long-term implanted device.

bridge to transplant: the process whereby a ventricular assist device is used to prevent death from heart failure until a donor heart can be found. At the time of transplant, the pump and diseased heart are both removed.

cannula: a plastic tube inserted into the heart or a blood vessel to carry blood or fluid.

capillaries: billions of microscopic single-cell-thick blood channels that exchange nutrients, oxygen, carbon dioxide, and metabolic by-products with the tissues of the body.

cardiac catheterization: a long fine-bore catheter is passed from the groin or wrist up into the heart or coronary arteries. Contrast medium is injected rapidly to demonstrate the internal anatomy of the heart or blood vessels. The catheter is also used to measure pressure within the chambers.

cardiac tamponade: a condition that occurs when blood or fluid accumulates within the pericardial sac under pressure, preventing the heart from filling.

cardiomyopathy: heart-muscle disease. There are several causes, which may be impossible to define, thus the term "idiopathic," meaning a disease of unknown cause. Can occur spontaneously in all age groups, after pregnancy, or from poisoning with alcohol or other toxic substances. Causes chronic heart failure.

cardioplegia: a cold (39.2°F) clear or blood-based solution infused into the coronary arteries to stop and protect the heart in a flaccid state during surgery with the heart-lung machine. Usually contains a high concentration of potassium. At the end of the repair, the heart is re-animated by restoring normal coronary blood flow.

cardiopulmonary bypass (CPB): process whereby the patient's blood is diverted away from the heart and lungs for the duration of the surgical repair. Contact of the patient's blood with the synthetic surfaces in the pump-oxygenator system elicits an inflammatory response. This limits the safe duration of blood–foreign surface interaction. The longer the procedure, the more damaging is the whole-body inflammatory response.

CentriMag ventricular assist device: an external, magnetically levitated, centrifugal blood pump widely used for temporary circulatory support. Now marketed by Thoratec for use in cardiogenic shock.

chronic heart failure: the left ventricle fails gradually but inexorably due to a number of conditions, the commonest being coronary artery disease. Causes severe breathlessness and fatigue. Conveys a high mortality rate after two years.

congenital heart disease: heart deformity that the patient is born with (e.g., atrial septal defect, ventricular septal defect, dextrocardia).

coronary artery bypass grafts: operation to bypass the narrowing of the heart's own arteries, using pieces of the patient's chest-wall arteries, forearm arteries, or leg veins.

coronary artery disease: gradual narrowing of the coronary arteries by atheroma. These fatty, cholesterol-based plaques are prone to rupture when they suddenly occlude the vessel, which then clots (coronary thrombosis).

CT scan: X-ray-based three-dimensional imaging of the chest and heart. By adding contrast medium, the coronary arteries can be shown in detail.

deoxygenated blood: bluish blood leaving the tissues and returning to the right heart, now low in oxygen and carrying carbon dioxide to be expelled by the lungs. See also *oxygenated blood*.

diastole: relaxation and filling phase of the ventricles.

echocardiogram: non-invasive ultrasound examination of the heart chambers.

electrocautery: the electrical instrument used to cut through tissues and simultaneously coagulate blood vessels to stop bleeding.

endocarditis: bacterial infection that can destroy the heart valves.

extra-corporeal membrane oxygenation (ECMO): circuit outside the body with blood pump and long-term oxygenator (lasting days), used for temporary circulatory support in acute heart failure or severe lung failure. Attached to the body by percutaneous (through the skin) cannulation of the blood vessels to the leg. Usually functions as a bridge to a longer-term pump or transplantation.

heart-lung machine: circuit outside the body to keep the patient alive while the heart is stopped for repair. Contains a mechanical blood pump and a short-term (lasting hours) complex gas exchange mechanism known as the oxygenator (artificial lung). Other pumps are used for suction of blood into the reservoir and for delivery of cardioplegia fluid to stop the heart.

HeartMate left ventricular assist device: a large, pulsatile, implantable pump, now obsolete, widely used for bridge to transplant in the 1990s. The first device to be implanted on a permanent basis. Thoratec went on to produce a successful rotary blood pump for permanent use.

heart transplant: removal of the patient's diseased and failing heart, then replacement with an organ from a brain-dead donor.

heart valve replacement: removal of a diseased heart valve, then replacement with a prosthetic valve. Prosthetic valves can be biological (e.g., pig's valve) or mechanical (e.g., pyrolytic carbon tilting disc valves).

hypertension: high blood pressure that makes the heart work too hard. The level depends upon tone in the peripheral arteries. Can be very high (>200/120) and cause heart failure or stroke.

hypotension: low blood pressure (<90/60). Can be caused by blood loss or left ventricular failure. When pressure falls below 60/40 the patient is in shock and needs urgent resuscitation, and the kidneys cease to produce urine.

intra-aortic balloon pump (IABP): long, sausage-shaped balloon that is inserted into the aorta. When inflated in diastole and deflated during systole, it serves to lower the resistance against which the left ventricle has to pump. Used to support the left ventricle when it is struggling to cope. Ineffective in shock states when the blood pressure or blood volume is low.

Jarvik 2000: thumb-sized rotary blood pump that is inserted into the failing heart on a long-term basis. A long-term "off the shelf" solution for severe heart failure. The longest implant exceeds eight years.

left atrium: collecting chamber for blood returning to the heart from the lungs. The blood then passes through the mitral valve into the left ventricle. See also *right atrium*.

left ventricle: powerful, thick-walled conical chamber that pumps blood through the aortic valve and around the body. See also *right ventricle*.

left ventricular assist device (LVAD): mechanical blood pump to maintain the circulation and rest the ventricles when the heart fails catastrophically. The cannulas are inserted into the chambers of the heart. There are inexpensive temporary external devices suitable for several weeks of support in acute heart failure (e.g., CentriMag or Berlin Heart). The small, implantable but very expensive high-speed rotary blood pumps (e.g., Jarvik 2000) can be used for as long as ten years in chronic heart failure. As such, the long-term LVADs offer an off-the-shelf alternative to heart transplantation.

magnetic resonance imaging (MRI): non-invasive (without X-ray), detailed study of an organ's (e.g., heart) morphology.

metabolic derangement: consequence of poor tissue blood flow. Arteries to the muscles clamp down, and the tissues produce lactic acid and other toxic metabolites.

mitral stenosis: narrowing of the mitral valve between left atrium and left ventricle caused by rheumatic fever. Flow through the valve is restricted, causing breathlessness and chronic fatigue.

myocardial infarction: death of part of the heart when a coronary artery occludes suddenly. Dead muscle is replaced by scar.

myocarditis: virus infection of the heart muscle itself, causing the heart to fail.

oxygenated blood: bright-red blood saturated with oxygen and pumped around the body by the left ventricle. See also *deoxygenated blood*.

perfusionist: technician who controls the heart-lung machine and ventricular assist devices.

pericardium: fibrous sac that surrounds the heart. Can be used as patch material in the heart. Calf pericardium is used to make bio-prosthetic heart valves.

pulmonary artery: large, thin-walled vessel that carries blood from the right ventricle to the lungs. It bifurcates into right and left pulmonary arteries.

pulmonary edema: "water on the lungs" that occurs when the left ventricle fails. Is often frothy and blood-stained.

pulmonary veins: four veins leaving the lungs to bring blood back to the heart.

reperfusion: the process whereby blood is allowed back into the coronary arteries and heart muscle following cardioplegia and cardiac arrest during surgery. The heart is re-animated and begins to beat again.

rheumatic fever: autoimmune condition triggered by a streptococcus bacterial infection that damages the heart valves and joints. Very common cause of valve disease in the pre-antibiotic era.

right atrium: collecting chamber for blood returning to the heart from the body via the veins. The blood then passes through the tricuspid valve into the right ventricle. See also *left atrium*.

right ventricle: crescent-shaped pumping chamber that propels blood through the pulmonary valve and to the lungs. See also *left ventricle*.

shock: condition when the heart cannot continue to supply sufficient blood and oxygen to the tissues. Cardiogenic shock occurs after a heart attack. Hemorrhagic shock follows profuse bleeding of two liters or more.

systole: phase of the heart cycle when the ventricles contract to expel blood.

veins: thinner-walled vessels that return blood to the heart.

vena cava: large vein entering the right atrium. The superior vena cava drains the upper part of the body; the inferior vena cava drains the lower half.

Index

Courtesy of John Radcliffe Hospital

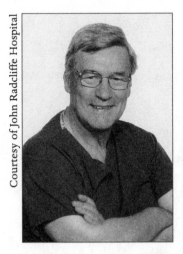

STEPHEN WESTABY is a pioneer in artificial-heart technology and served as consultant cardiac surgeon at the John Radcliffe Hospital, Oxford. He was a member of the American Association of Thoracic Surgeons, the Society of Thoracic Surgeons US, and a fellow of the American College of Cardiology. Westaby received the prestigious Ray C. Fish Award for Scientific Achievement from the Texas Heart Institute and the Vladimir Bourokovsky Gold Medal from the Bakoulev Institute, Moscow. He lives in Oxford, United Kingdom.